THAMES VALLEY EMERGENCY SERVICE VEHICLES

GERAINT H. ROBERTS

AMBERLEY

This book is dedicated to my late father, Ray
'You often said I should write a book'

Front cover above: Three Thames Valley Police vehicles (Volvo XC90 Armed Response Vehicle, Ford Mondeo Dog Unit and Vauxhall Movano Personnel Carrier) seen in Windsor (Berkshire) on the day after the coronation of King Charles III in May 2023.

Front cover below: Lined up outside the front of Rewley Road Fire Station in Oxford one evening in April 2024 were three Oxfordshire Fire and Rescue Service, Volvo chassis appliances: Water Tender Ladder, Hydraulic Platform and another Water Tender Ladder.

Back cover top left: A South Central Ambulance Service, Fiat Ducato Emergency Ambulance and a Dacia Duster Dynamic Response Vehicle attending a call in Winterbrook, just south of Wallingford (Oxfordshire), in November 2023.

Back cover top right: Two of National Highways, Mercedes Sprinter Incident Units attending a diesel spill on the northbound A34 at Chilton (Oxfordshire), in May 2024.

Back cover below: Two of National Highways Traffic Officer hybrid vehicles based at the Chieveley Out-Station in Berkshire (Volvo XC90 and BMW X5), photographed on a very wet day in September 2024. Many thanks to National Highways for arranging a surprise photo opportunity on what is sometimes referred to on the internet as a secret slip road on the eastbound carriageway of the M4 in Berkshire.

First published 2025

Amberley Publishing
The Hill, Stroud
Gloucestershire, GL5 4EP

www.amberley-books.com

ISBN 978 1 3981 2295 6 (print)
ISBN 978 1 3981 2296 3 (ebook)

British Library Cataloguing in Publication Data.
A catalogue record for this book is available from the British Library.

Origination by Amberley Publishing.
Printed in the UK.

Appointed GPSR EU Representative: Easy Access System Europe Oü, 16879218
Address: Mustamäe tee 50, 10621, Tallinn, Estonia
Contact Details: gpsr.requests@easproject.com, +358 40 500 3575

About the Author

With an interest in the emergency services starting as a child, Geraint has photographed emergency vehicles from above the Arctic Circle to New Zealand. A lifelong resident of Oxfordshire, he has worked in radiological protection for over thirty years, including emergency planning, participating in and planning exercises, and providing training for police, fire and rescue and NHS staff (A&E and ambulance service, including HART personnel). He is married with two children. He has had articles on emergency vehicles and the emergency services published in magazines in the UK and Germany and has had photographs published in four books. This is the first book he has written.

Introduction

The Thames Valley can be defined in more than one way. However, for the purposes of this book, it is the area covered by the Thames Valley Police; specifically, the three ceremonial counties of Berkshire, Buckinghamshire and Oxfordshire. The Thames Valley is located in the north-west corner of the South East region of England and borders the London, East of England, East Midlands, West Midlands and South West regions. More information on the Thames Valley is included in the introductions to each chapter.

Having an almost lifelong interest in the emergency services, my intention of writing this book was to feature both current and previous vehicles, highlighting as much as possible the wide variety of roles, vehicle types, manufacturers and liveries used by the emergency services in the Thames Valley since the 1980s, including the lesser-seen vehicles, such as driver training and support units. Also, to emphasise the not-so-well-known emergency services and supporting organisations, both professional and volunteer, civilian and military, publically funded and charitable, that operate in the Thames Valley in addition to the ambulance service, fire and rescue services and police forces.

The work of the emergency services, not just across the Thames Valley or the United Kingdom but throughout the world, can be unpredictable, difficult, stressful, dangerous, exhausting, emotional, thankless and violent – it is a sad reflection on some parts of society in the UK that we now have a specific criminal offence of common assault or battery that is committed against an emergency worker (Assaults on Emergency Workers (Offences) Act 2018). However, emergency services personnel are caring, compassionate, thoughtful and helpful; I've always been appreciative of the times when they have been prepared to take a few minutes out of their busy shifts to allow photographs to be taken of a vehicle and to answer questions.

Some of the locations featured in this book are not normally accessible to the public and permission to visit them to take photographs was obtained in advance. Many of the photographs were taken in public places or at events and locations where the public was admitted (e.g. open days) and the aim has always been to photograph vehicles without identifiable members of the public or emergency services personnel in the photographs. Some vehicles were photographed attending incidents but none of the photographs show people being arrested, the injured or people who have been rescued. While no unmarked vehicles are included in this book, at the request of some of the police forces, certain vehicles have their registrations obscured and for some organisations only historic vehicles are included.

Unless stated otherwise, all photographs were taken by me between 1986 and 2024, using a variety of film and digital cameras and mobile phones. The text and captions have been written based on my own knowledge of the emergency services, notes taken by me and information provided at events and by other knowledgeable individuals; and my research using books and the internet. All information was checked and accurate at the time of writing and any mistakes are my own.

Chapter 1
Ambulance Services

Nearly all of the Thames Valley is covered by one of the National Health Service's (NHS) ten regional ambulance services in England: The South Central Ambulance Service (SCAS), which was formed on 1 July 2006 by merging the Hampshire, Oxfordshire and Royal Berkshire ambulance services and the Buckinghamshire area of the Two Shires Ambulance Service (the Northamptonshire area became part of the East Midlands Ambulance Service).

Becoming a NHS Foundation Trust in 2012, SCAS provides a range of emergency, urgent care and non-emergency healthcare services, along with a commercial logistics service, to around 3.8 million people in Berkshire, Buckinghamshire, most of Hampshire and most of Oxfordshire, as well as non-emergency patient transport services in Surrey and Sussex (from April 2025, a private contractor will provide the patient transport service in the NHS Buckinghamshire, Oxfordshire, Berkshire West and Frimley areas). A small part of north-east Hampshire is covered by the South East Coast Ambulance Service and a very small part of south-west Oxfordshire is covered by the South Western Ambulance Service.

SCAS employs over 4,000 staff with over 1,000 volunteer community and co-responders, attending over half a million incidents per year.

Over 1,300 vehicles, ranging from double-crewed emergency ambulances, single-crewed rapid response vehicles, patient transport vehicles, four wheel drive vehicles, officers' cars, command vehicles, equipment vehicles, specialist response vehicles, training vehicles, vans and trucks, plus new electric vehicles, form the fleet.

Staff are based at around thirty locations, including headquarters (Northern at Bicester, Oxfordshire, and Southern at Otterbourne, Hampshire), control centres (Bicester and Otterbourne), Hazardous Area Response Team (Eastleigh, Hampshire), training centres (e.g. Newbury, Berkshire), vehicle workshops (Milton, Oxfordshire, and Nursling, Hampshire), resource centres (e.g. Bracknell, Berkshire), ambulance stations (e.g. Kidlington, Oxfordshire) and patient transport service bases (e.g. Maids Norton, Buckinghamshire), plus there are numerous standby points (e.g. Abingdon, Oxfordshire), in two areas (Northern and Southern), covering an area of around 9,100 square kilometres (around 3,500 square miles).

SCAS works closely with two air ambulance charities, the Hampshire and Isle of Wight and the Thames Valley air ambulances.

In addition, a number of military, private and volunteer ambulance services operate in the Thames Valley area. Some of these are under contract to the NHS, including the British Emergency Ambulance Response Service, which operates a high-dependency patient transport service between the Neonatal Intensive Care and Paediatric Intensive Care units at the John Radcliffe Hospital in Oxford and the Princess Anne Hospital in Southampton.

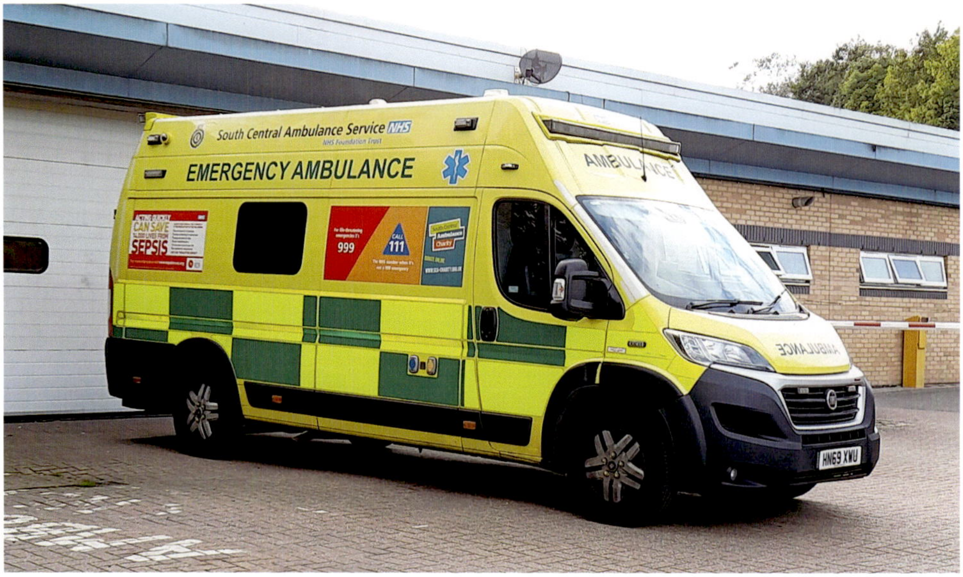

Large numbers of Emergency Ambulances built by WAS on Fiat Ducato chassis, fitted with Euro 6 emission standard diesel engines, have been placed in service with NHS ambulance services in recent years. HN69 XWU (2019) was seen outside the North Oxfordshire Resource Centre in the village of Adderbury, south of Banbury, in Oxfordshire, on an August evening in 2023.

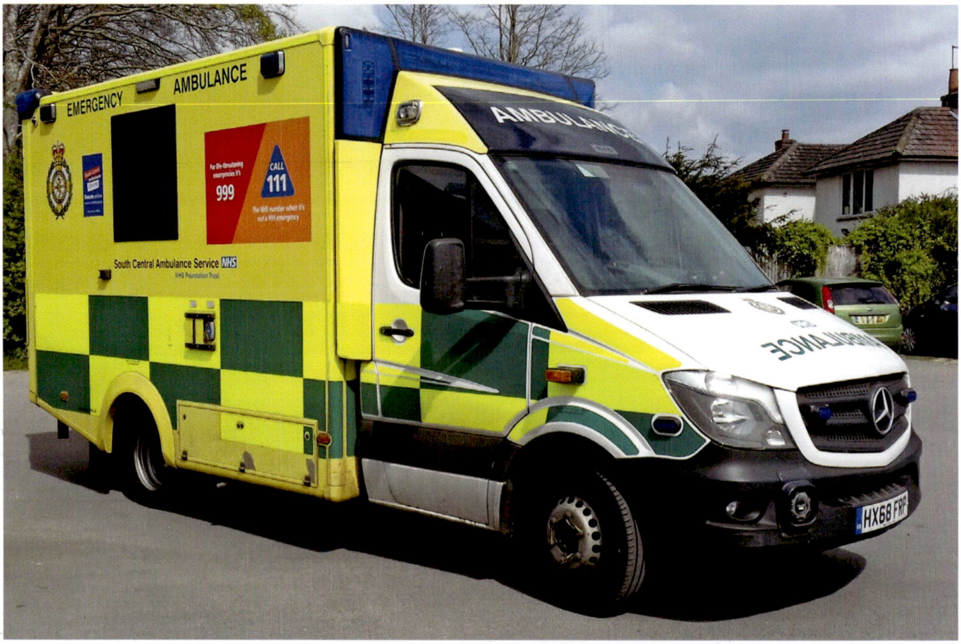

An unexpected visitor to the venue of the author's daughter's birthday party in April 2022 was this EA from Oxford Ambulance Station. Call-sign North Ambulance Four Two Four was sent to a minor incident in Cholsey in Oxfordshire but the casualty had been taken to hospital by other means. HX68 FRP is a 2018 Mercedes Sprinter chassis bodied by WAS; the German ambulance builder has its UK base in Burton-upon-Trent, Staffordshire.

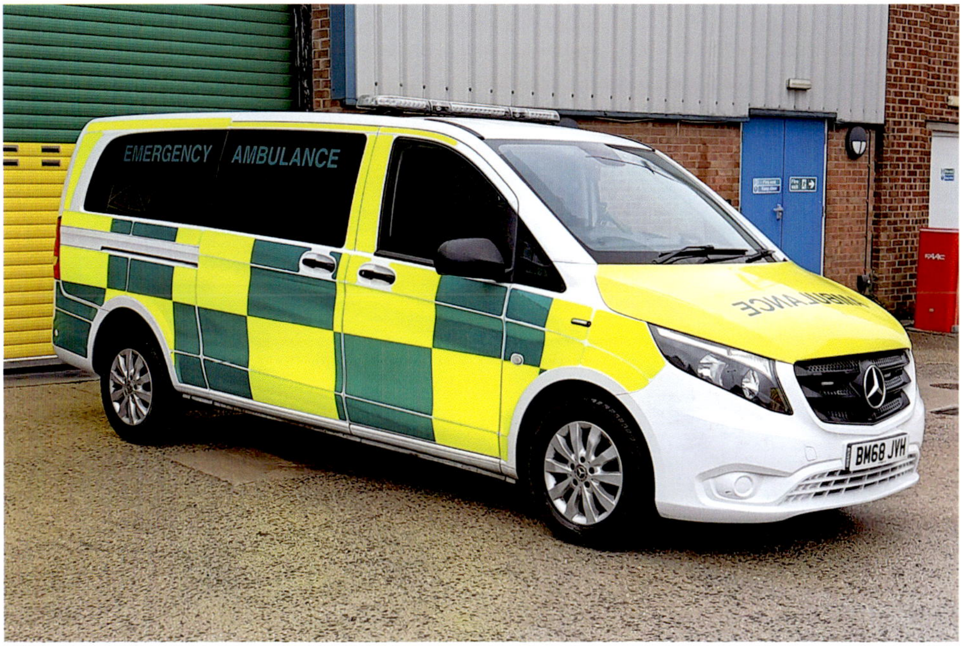

A 'one-off' in the training fleet at SCAS's Newbury Education Centre in Berkshire is BM68 JVH (2019), a LWB Mercedes Vito. The Newbury Education Centre provides recruit courses, refresher training, specialist courses and driver training. The driver training fleet includes a range of Mercedes van-based vehicles, Fiat van-based vehicles and Skoda Superb estate cars.

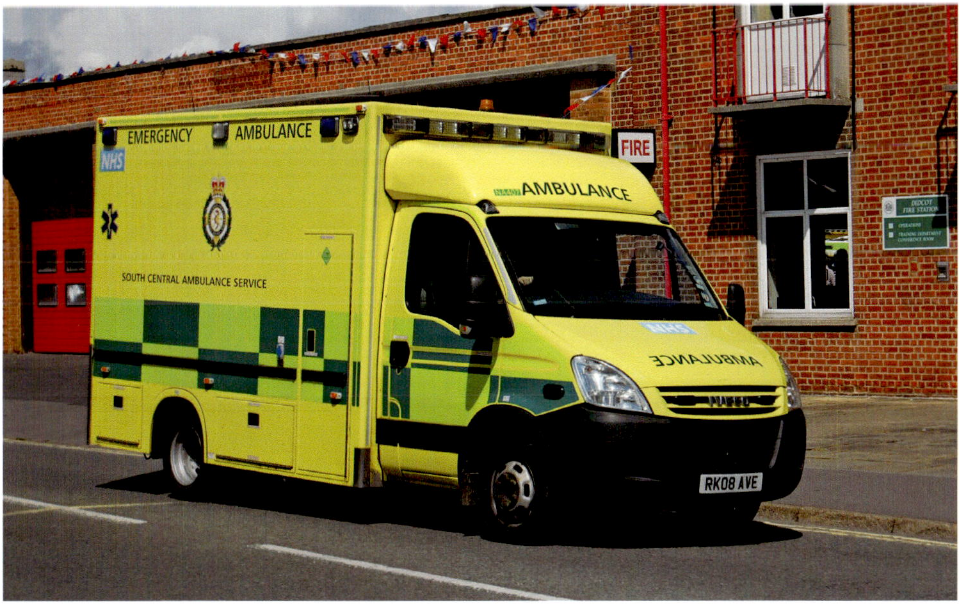

An ex-Royal Berkshire Ambulance Service, Emergency Ambulance, call-sign North Ambulance Four Zero Seven, RK08 AVE (2008) was seen about to turn into the drill yard at Didcot Fire Station in Oxfordshire for an open day in June 2012. This is a second generation version of the Iveco Daily with the restyled cab, built at Iveco's plant at Suzzara in northern Italy.

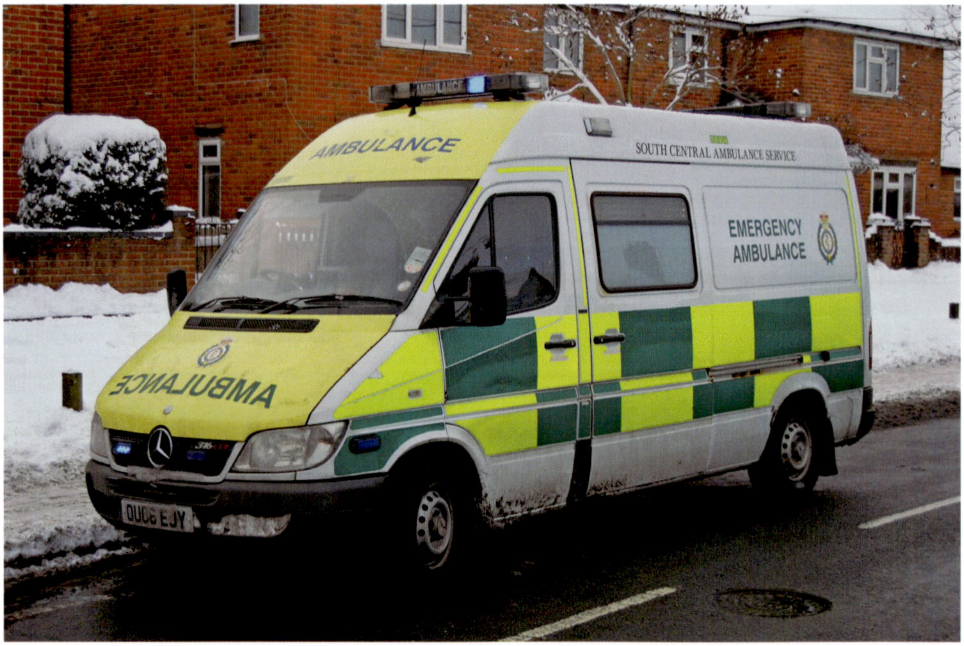

OU06 EJY (2006) was an ex-Oxfordshire Ambulance Service, Mercedes Sprinter 316CDi/ Wilker, Emergency Ambulance. Based at Didcot, call-sign North Ambulance Four Zero Four was seen attending an emergency call in nearby Wallingford in the snow just before Christmas 2010. Emergency Ambulances are also referred to as double-crewed ambulances.

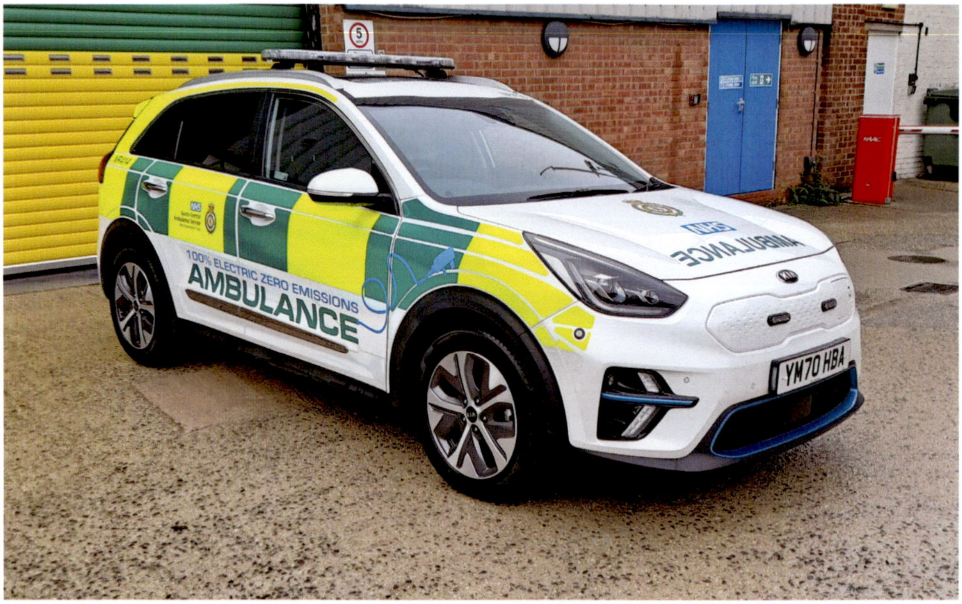

YM70 HBA (2021), call-sign NR414, is one of two electric-powered Kia eNero Rapid Response Vehicles (RRV) in the SCAS fleet, which was seen at SCAS's Newbury Education Centre on 6 September 2024. The other one of the pair is based at Kidlington in Oxfordshire and is operational with a specialist paramedic team.

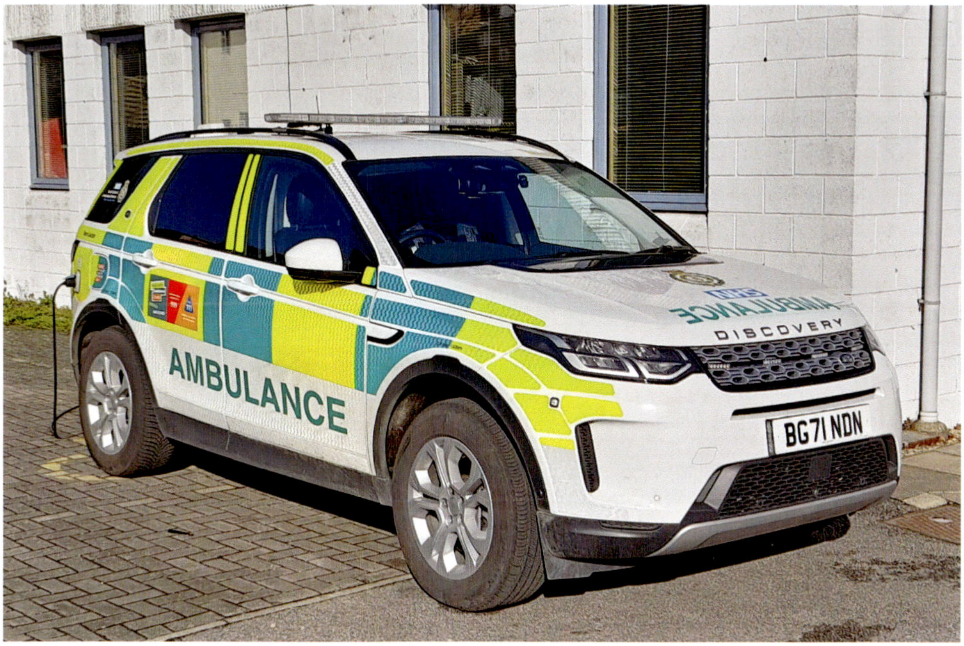

SCAS has used the Land Rover Discovery 4x4 for many years. The latest model to be used is the Discovery Sport SD. An example is BG71 NDN (2021), call-sign NT498, a Team Leader's Vehicle seen outside the Didcot Resource Centre when just a few months old in March 2022. Team Leaders can also act as Operations Managers at incidents.

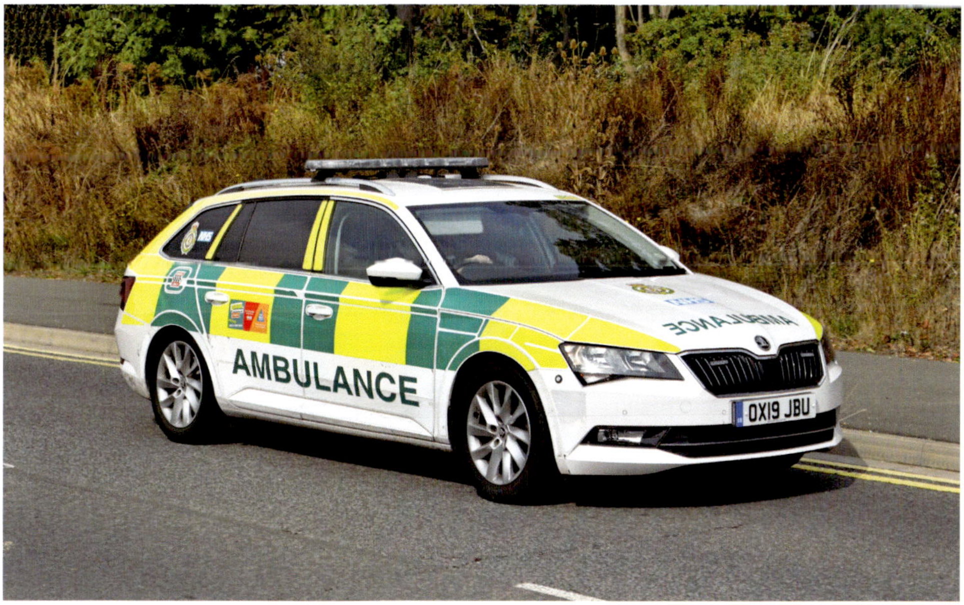

Another type of vehicle which has been placed in service in large numbers with NHS ambulances services is the Skoda Octavia and Superb estate car, for use as RRVs. OX19 JBU, call-sign NR311, is a 2019 Skoda Superb estate, which was seen passing Aylesbury Fire Station in Buckinghamshire in September 2022.

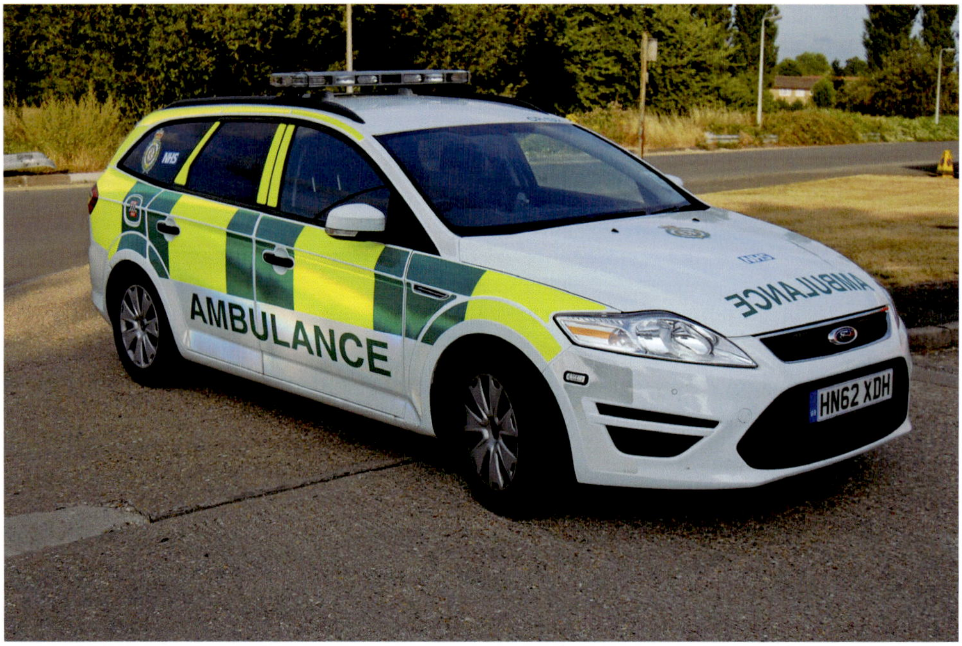

HN62 XDH (2012) is a 2-litre diesel engine Ford Mondeo estate car, seen parked outside Maidenhead Fire Station in Berkshire on a July evening in 2013. Call-sign CR132. As with the Skoda Superb, some of the SCAS Mondeos had solar panels on the roof to help keep electrical equipment charged.

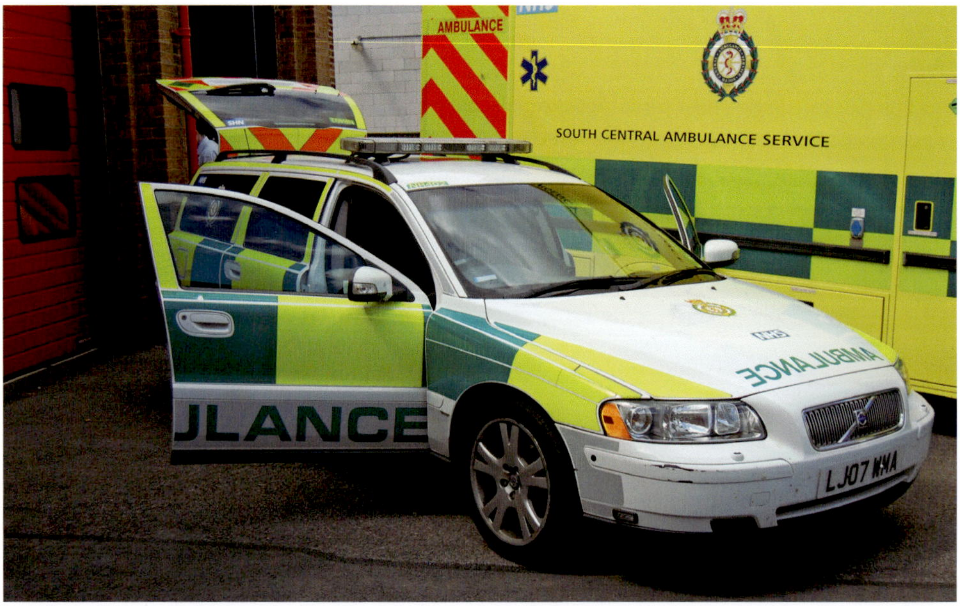

On display at Didcot Fire Station open day in 2012 was LJ07 MWA (2007), a Volvo V70 estate, RRV, call-sign NR402. The ambulance and fire stations are located next to each other on Broadway, the main road through the centre of Didcot, which is the largest town in South Oxfordshire and has expanded rapidly since the turn of the century.

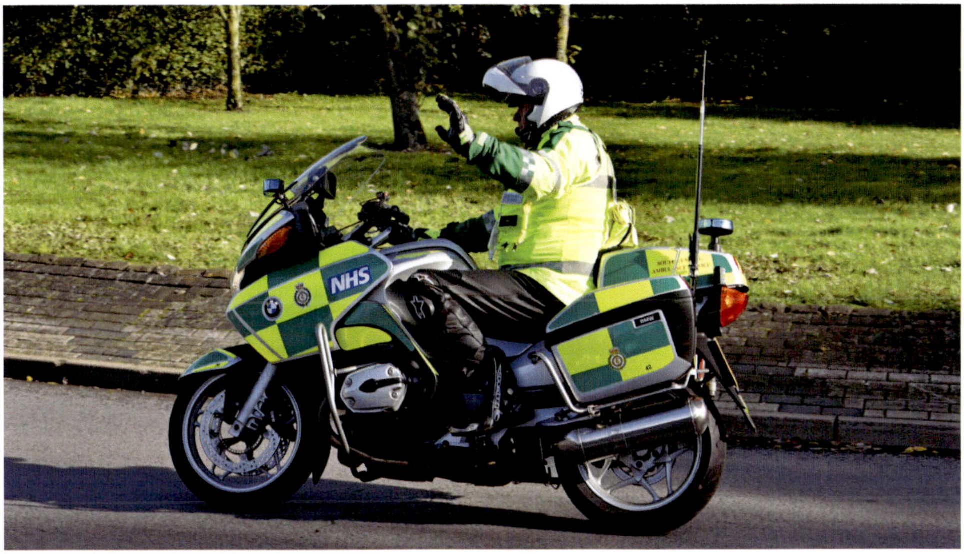

This ambulance officer was among 4,000 motorcyclists in the Ride of Respect 2019 from RAF Benson to Dalton Barracks (formerly RAF Abingdon) in memory of Thames Valley Police Constable Andrew Harper, who died on duty while attending a call to a burglary in West Berkshire in August 2019. PC Harper grew up in Wallingford and was a member of the Roads Policing Unit based at Abingdon Police Station. Seen negotiating the A4074/A4130 roundabout at Crowmarsh is a 2009 BMW R1200 RT (LF59 XSA), based in Reading.

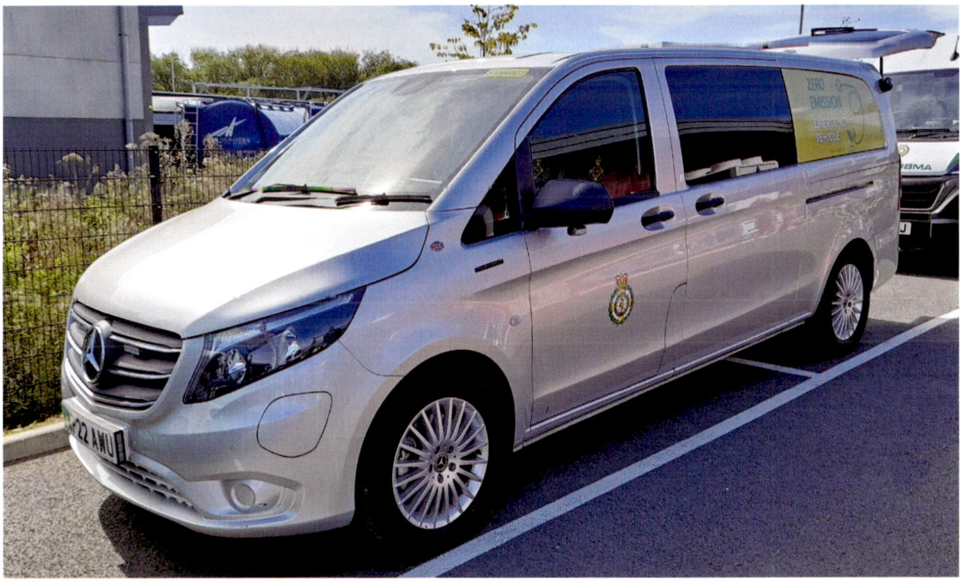

Seen at the West Ashland Blue Light Hub open day in 2023 was a visitor from SCAS's Southern Area. This discreetly marked electric vehicle is a Mental Health Response Unit, which responds to people who urgently require support for their mental health. WP22 AWU (2022) is a Mercedes Vito Electric converted by CVC. The vehicle provides a safe space for counselling and can also respond to Category A calls, carrying defibrillator, primary, secondary, paediatric, oxygen and entonox bags in the rear.

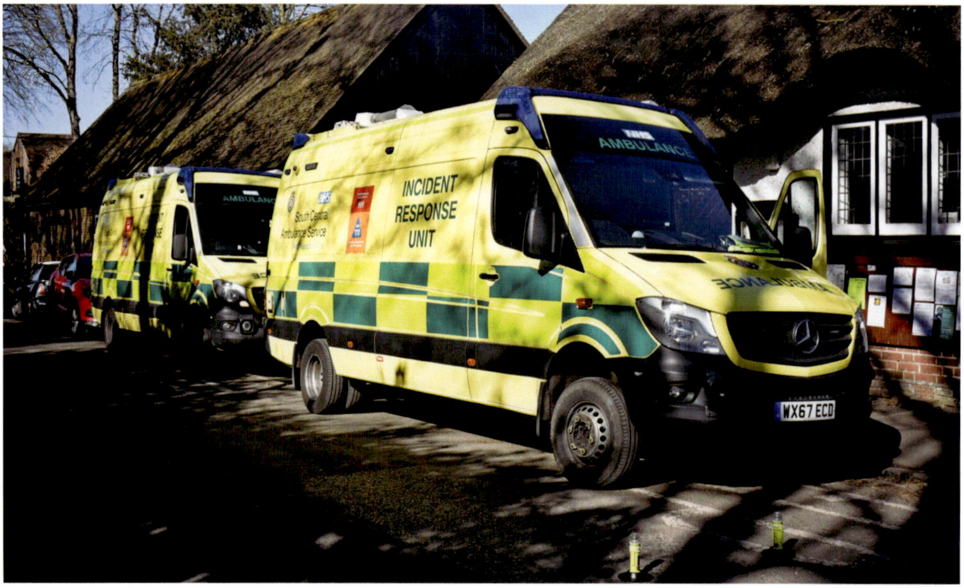

The late winter sun casts shadows on the sides of two SCAS Hazardous Area Response Team, Incident Response Unit, Mercedes Sprinter 4x4/WAS vehicles attending a Make Pumps Ten fire involving a thatched roof at Ewelme in South Oxfordshire on Sunday 27 February 2022. The four crew members had travelled 60 miles north from the HART base at Eastleigh in Hampshire. HART paramedics are trained in BA, working at height, water rescue and to work in the hot zone at hazmat, CBRN, USAR and firearms incidents.

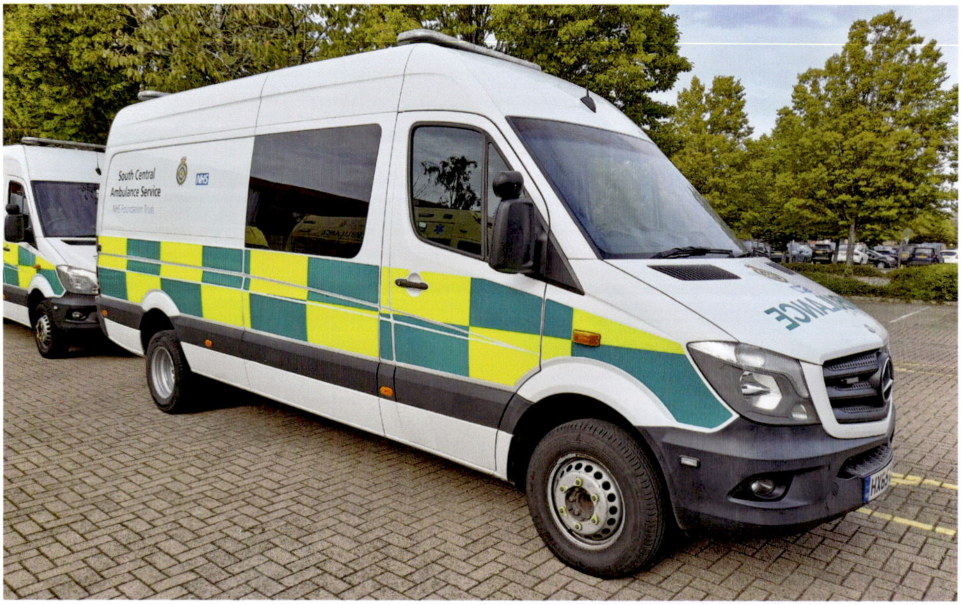

SCAS has several vehicles used for driver training, including ambulances, long wheel-base vans and crew-cab vehicles with box bodies. Some of the vehicles are plain white while others have the Battenberg livery. Photographed at SCAS's Northern HQ in Bicester in October 2023 was DTV02, a 2015 Mercedes Sprinter LWB combi van (HX65 UZB).

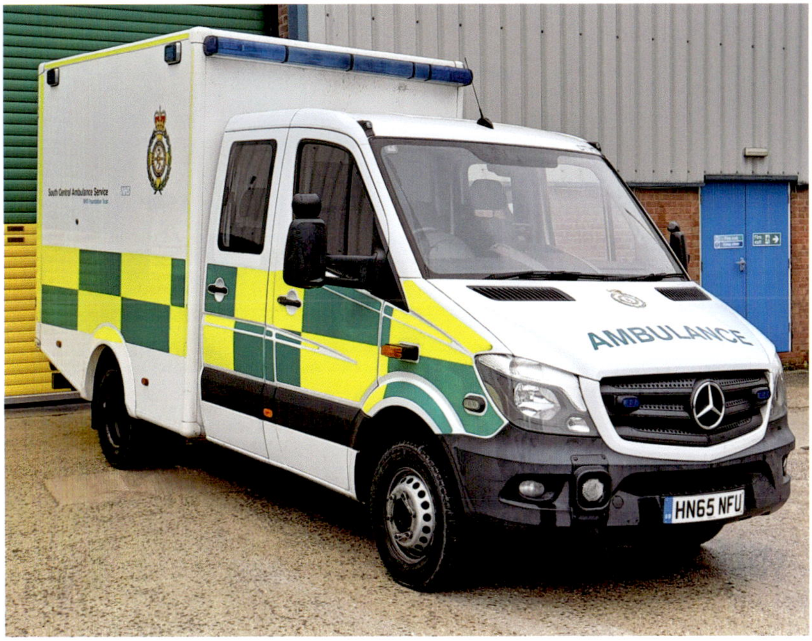

Another type of Driver Training Vehicle is this Mercedes Sprinter LWB crew cab with a box body built by WAS. HN65 NFU (2016), DTV17, is based at the Newbury Education Centre in Berkshire. Driver training courses are run at Bicester, Newbury and Southampton.

BUCKINGHAMSHIRE

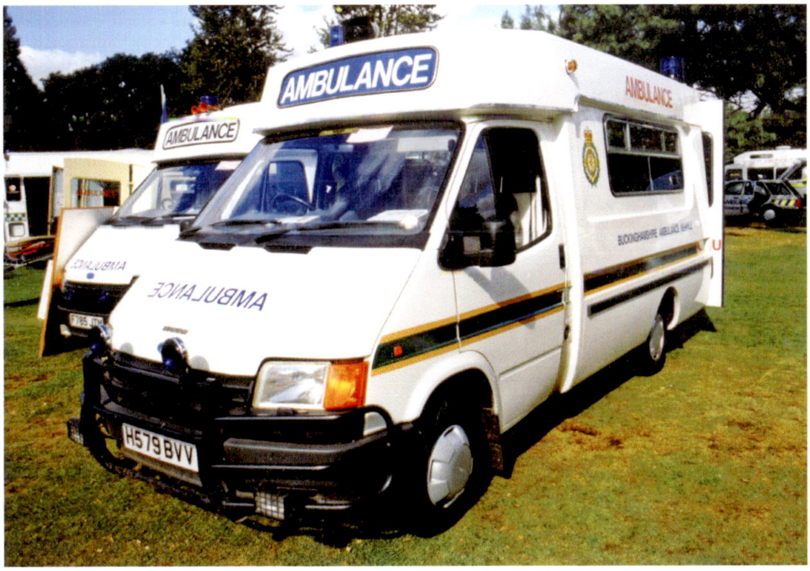

In the late 1980s/early 1990s, the newer ambulances in both Buckinghamshire and Oxfordshire had similar markings of dark green stripe with thin yellow stripes. H579 BVV (registered in Northampton in 1991) was a Ford Transit LWB chassis bodied by Mountain Range, a company based in Cheshire which also built fire appliances.

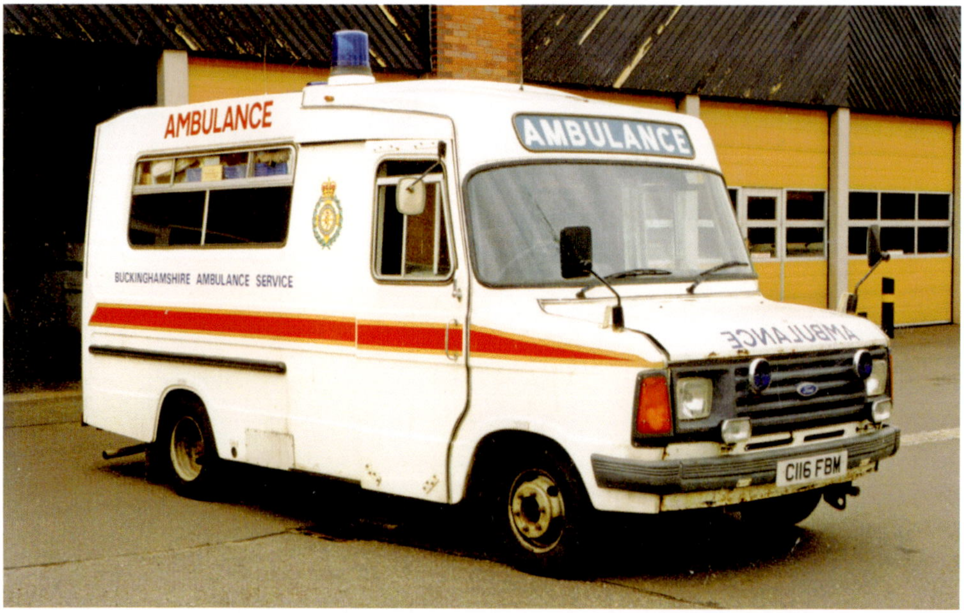

This Emergency Ambulance (registered in Luton in 1985) was a reserve when seen at Stoke Mandeville Ambulance Station on the south-eastern edge of Aylesbury, the county town of Buckinghamshire. This Ford Transit LWB chassis was bodied by Irish ambulance builder Hanlon, then based in County Longford.

TWO SHIRES

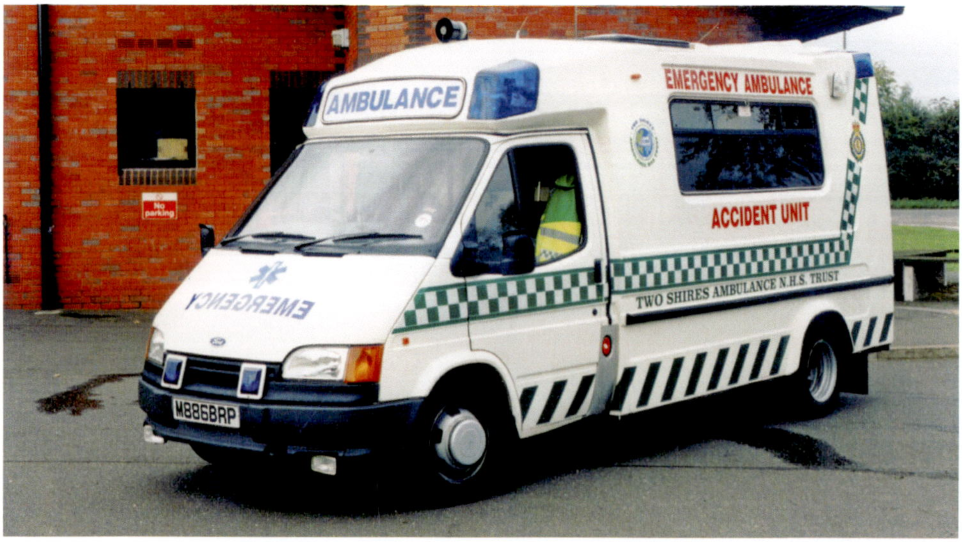

Also seen at Stoke Mandeville Ambulance Station was this 1994 Ford Transit/Wilker Emergency Ambulance/Accident Unit. These vehicles were some of the first EAs to be ordered by the then new Two Shires Ambulance Service, which was a merger of the Buckinghamshire and Northamptonshire Ambulance Services. Wilker is based in County Offaly, Ireland, and has its UK base in Sandbach, Cheshire.

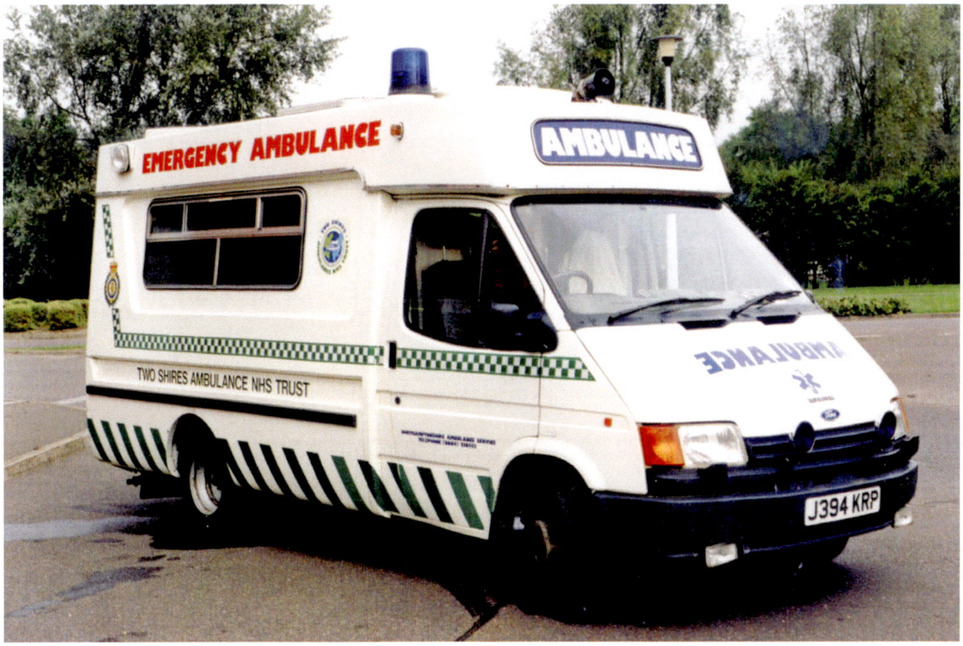

In addition to Buckinghamshire and Oxfordshire, the Northamptonshire Ambulance Service also bought Mountain Range-bodied EAs based on the Ford Transit LWB chassis. New in 1991, this vehicle was also seen at Stoke Mandeville Ambulance Station and still had Northamptonshire Ambulance Service lettering on the doors.

OXFORDSHIRE

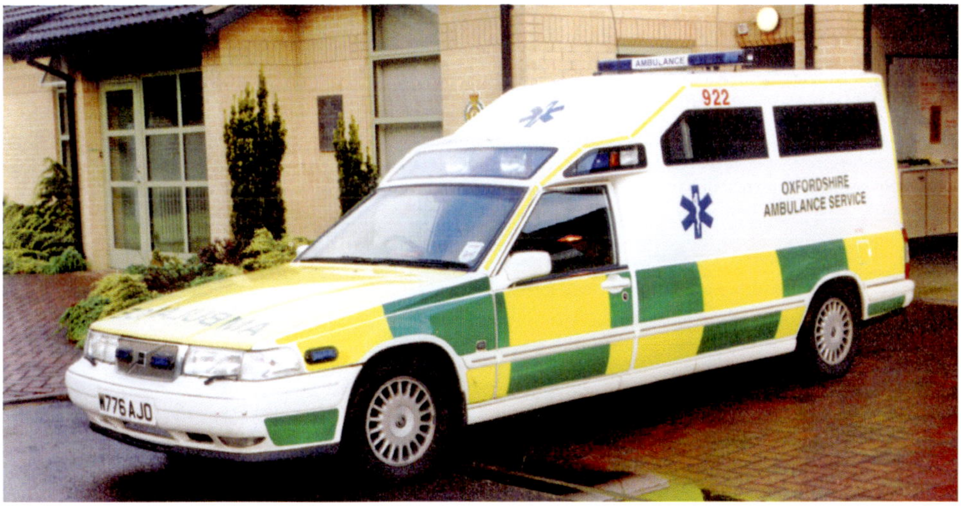

The Oxfordshire Ambulance Service was one of only a very few ambulances services, along with Shropshire and Wiltshire, to use fast Emergency Ambulances based on the Volvo V90 chassis bodied by Nilsson of Sweden, giving them a Scandinavian appearance. Call-sign Nine Two Two was based at Kidlington in the early 2000s, before being refurbished, repainted yellow and used as an events vehicle.

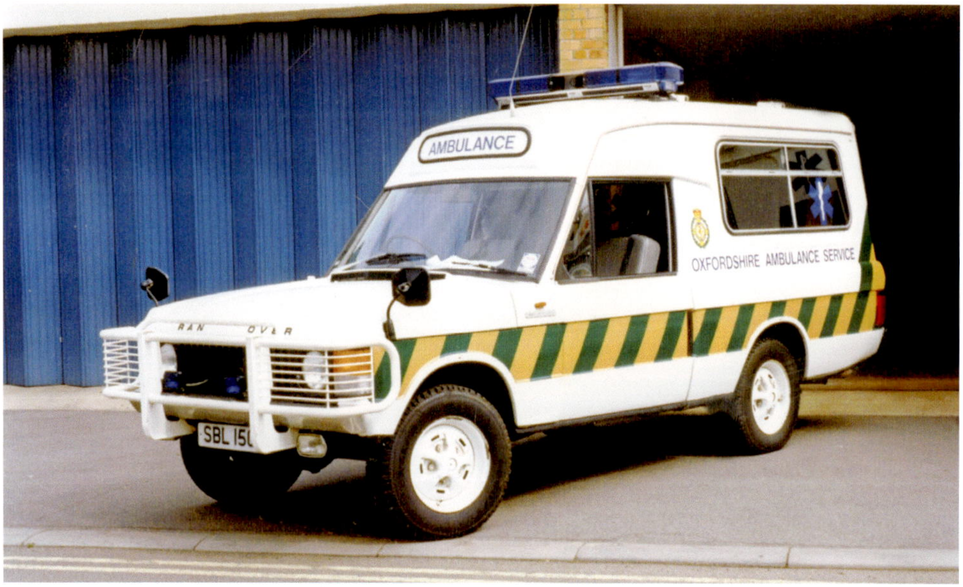

This Range Rover 4x4 ambulance started life as an Incident Control Unit. SBL 150M (1973) was previously fitted with a Stemlite lighting mast and a loudspeaker on the roof. Photographed outside the former Banbury Ambulance Station in the early 2000s, the site (next to Banbury Fire Station) was redeveloped for housing and replaced by a new North Oxfordshire Resource Centre in the village of Adderbury, south of Banbury, in 2006, just prior to the formation of the SCAS.

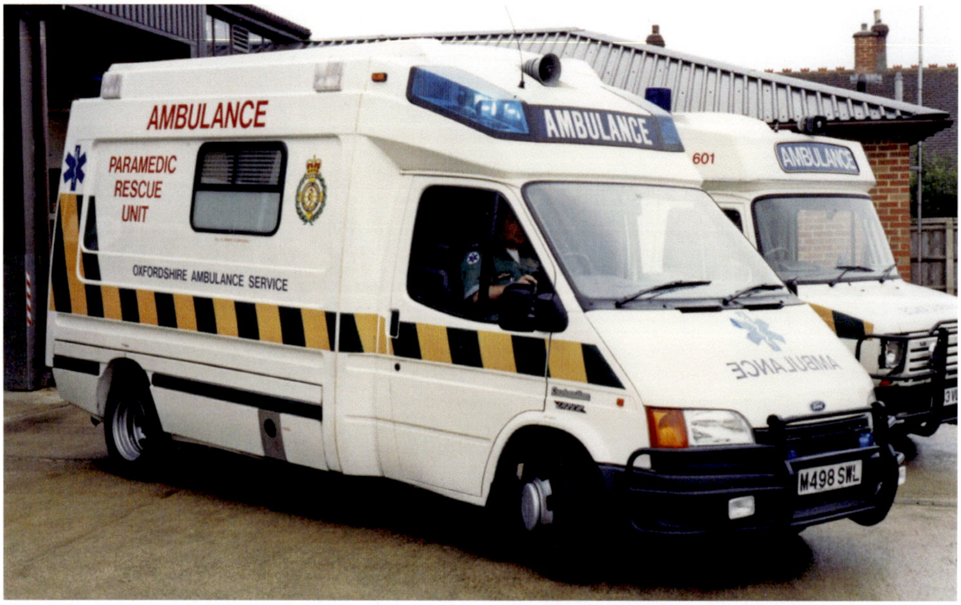

Prior to the introduction of the Battenberg livery, Oxfordshire Ambulance Service vehicles had diagonal dark green and gold stripes. Marked as a Paramedic Rescue Unit is this 1994 Ford Transit LWB chassis fitted with Customline's Lazer bodywork (M498 SWL) and seen at the former Wantage Ambulance Station in the late 1990s.

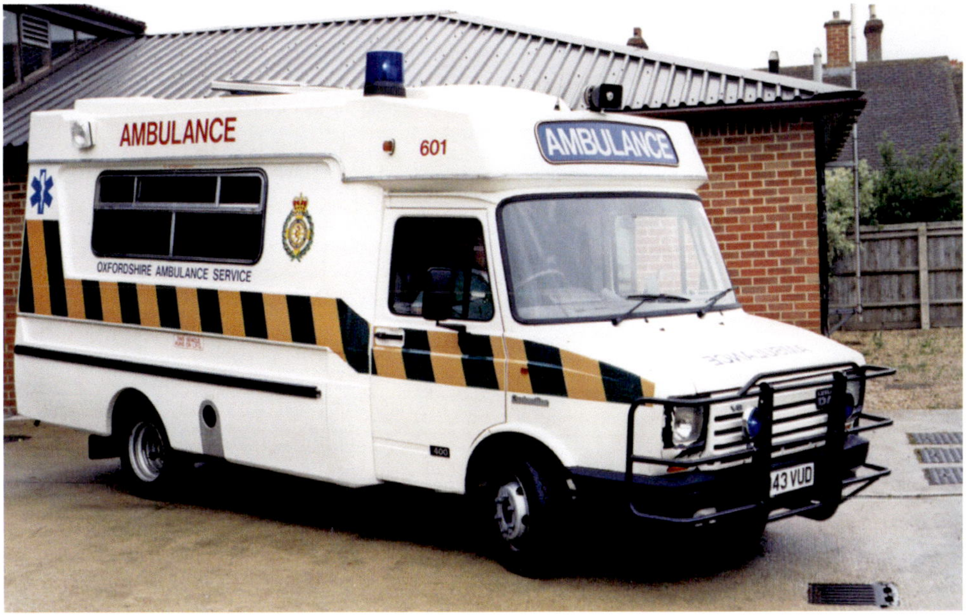

Call-sign Six Zero One was one of six Emergency Ambulances built by Customline on Leyland Daf 400 chassis, powered by V8 engines fuelled by liquefied petroleum gas (LPG). K943 VUD (1992) was also seen at Wantage where the then relatively newly built ambulance station was located behind Wantage Fire Station. The ambulance station site has since been redeveloped for housing.

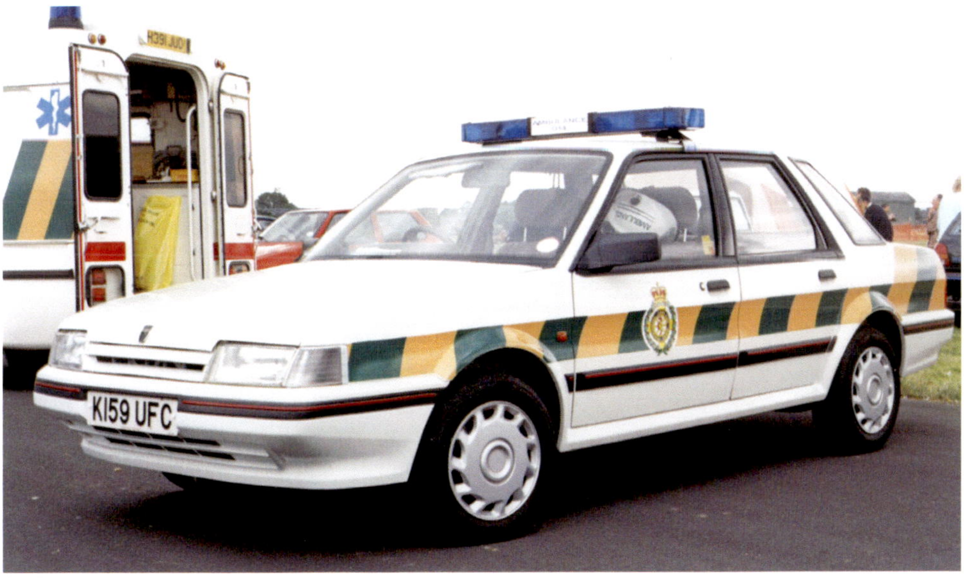

Attending an event in Abingdon in the mid-1990s was call-sign Zero One Four, one of five of a second batch of Rover Montego saloon cars, built locally at the Cowley plant in Oxford, which entered service as Officer's Cars in 1992 and were registered K156–160 UFC. Later, Vauxhall Cavalier saloons, Nissan Primera hatchbacks, Vauxhall Vectra hatchbacks and Skoda Octavia estates were used.

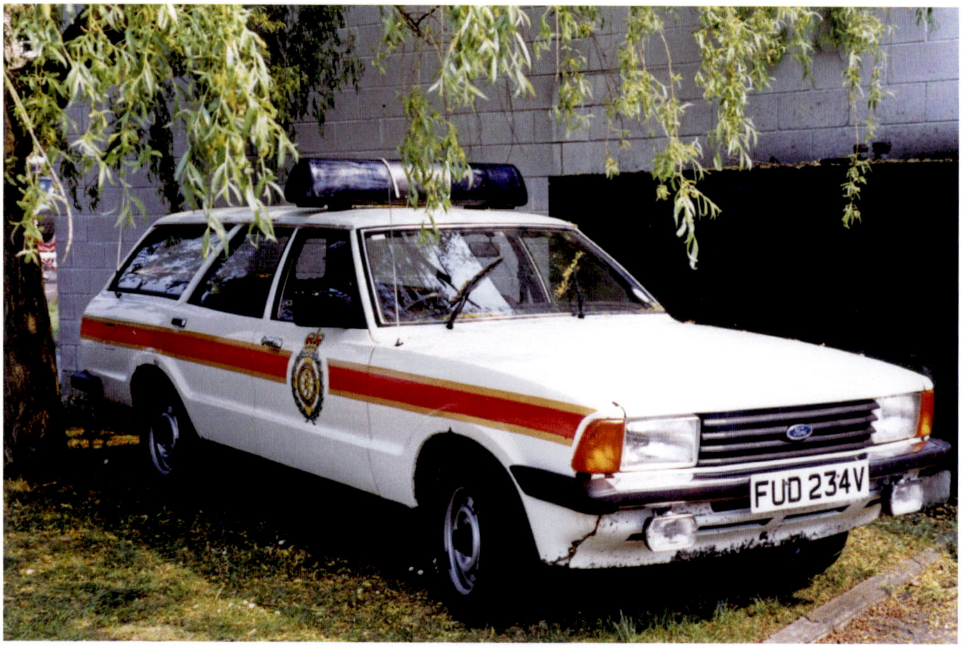

In July 1989, Didcot Fire Station and the neighbouring Didcot Ambulance Station (since renamed as Didcot Resource Centre) held a joint open day. Parked in the shade of a willow tree at the rear of the ambulance station was this Ford Cortina 1.6 estate Officer's Car, dating from 1980. These cars were replaced by a batch of G-reg Montego saloons at the end of 1989.

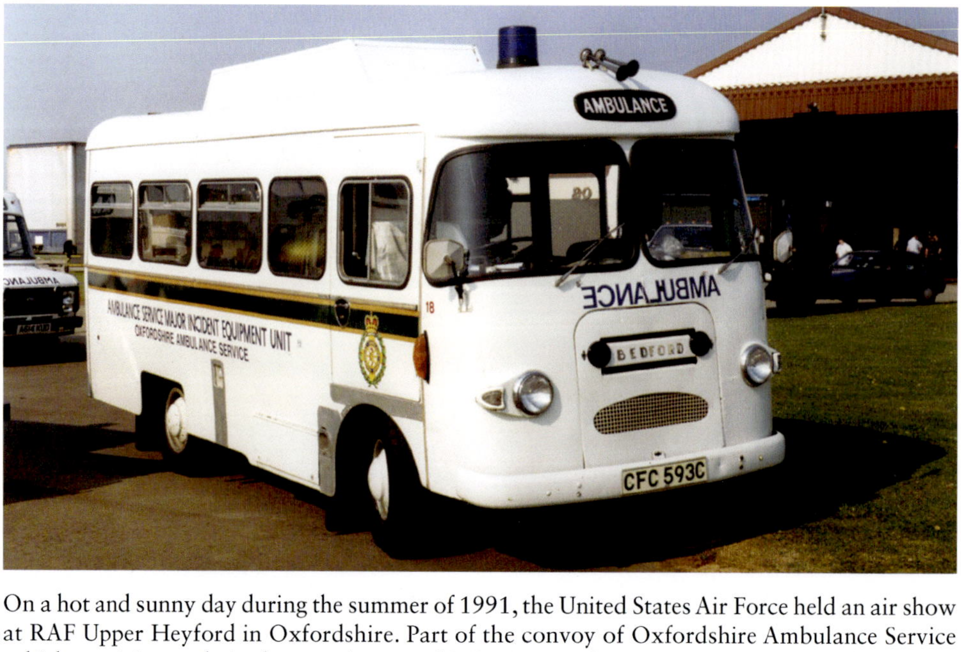

On a hot and sunny day during the summer of 1991, the United States Air Force held an air show at RAF Upper Heyford in Oxfordshire. Part of the convoy of Oxfordshire Ambulance Service vehicles arriving early in the morning was this Major Incident Equipment Unit. Understood to have been built as a coach on a Bedford chassis, this 1965-registered vehicle was refurbished and converted into its new role by the OAS workshop.

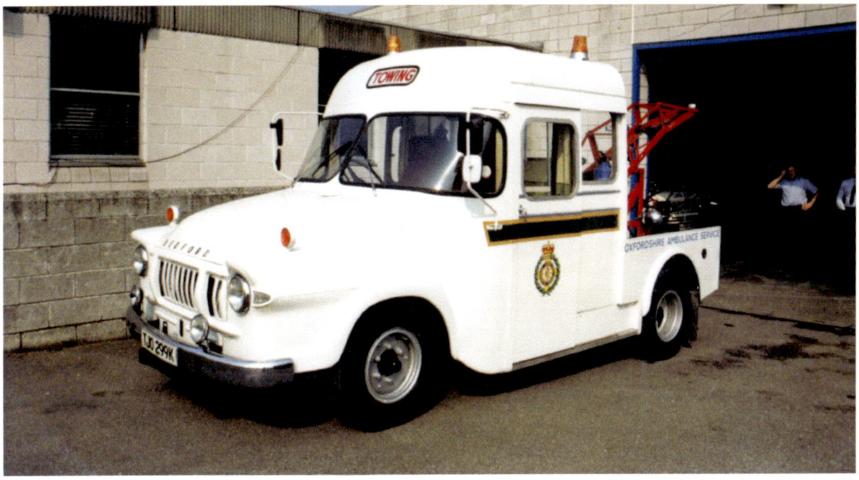

Seen on the forecourt of Didcot Ambulance Station in the early 1990s was the OAS's Breakdown Truck/Towing Vehicle. Originally built as an ambulance for the Oxford City and Oxfordshire County Joint Ambulance Service in 1971, most of the bodywork was removed and a crane mounted over the rear axle. As a result of the National Health Service Reorganisation Act 1973, responsibility for the provision of ambulance services passed from local authorities to the NHS in 1974.

ROYAL BERKSHIRE

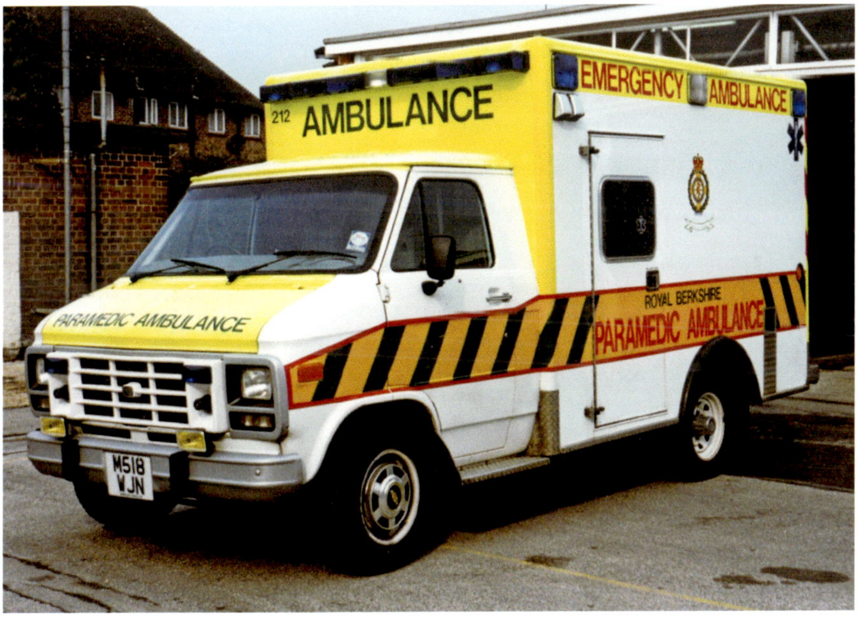

In the mid-1990s, the Royal Berkshire Ambulance Service (RBAS) operated a small number of American-style Emergency Ambulances, based on Chevrolet Chevy Van 30 chassis with Wheeled Coach box bodies; a similar EA was based on an American Ford Econovan chassis. Previously based at Reading Ambulance Station, with the call-sign Four One One, M518 WJN (1995) was seen at Newbury Ambulance Station in the late 1990s, with the call-sign having changed to Two One Two.

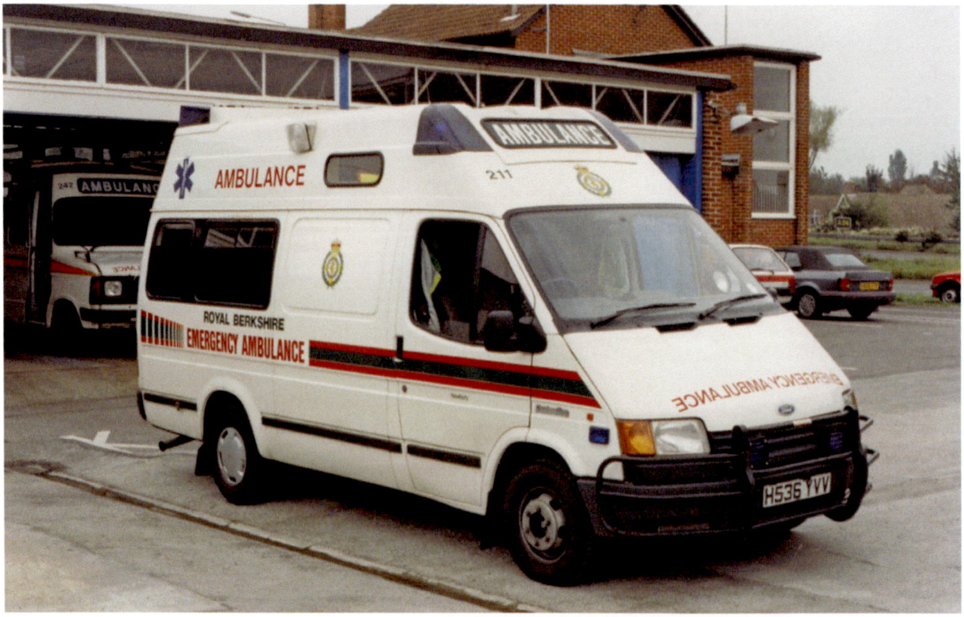

In the early 1990s, one of the Emergency Ambulances based at Newbury Ambulance Station was this 1990 Ford Transit LWB/Customline vehicle, call-sign Two One One. These vehicles were some of the first EAs to be fitted with intersection lights (small blue lights on the front wings) and scene lights (large floodlights on the top of each side). Later Ford Transits were bodied by French ambulance builder Collet.

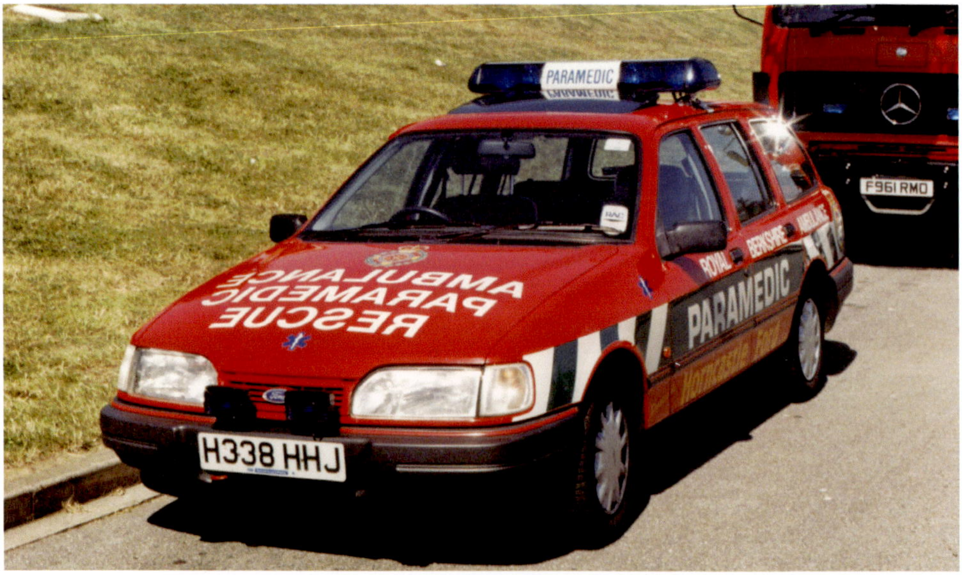

In September 1990 the author started a one day per week course at Reading College of Art and Technology and on the first day was surprised at seeing a red-liveried paramedic car passing the college on blues. H338 HHJ, a 1990 Ford Sierra 1.8-litre turbo diesel estate (call-sign Papa Mike One), was seen attending a fire in Reading. This was the first RRV in the RBAS fleet and was replaced by a Ford Sierra hatchback in a white livery. (Photo: Ivan Barefield)

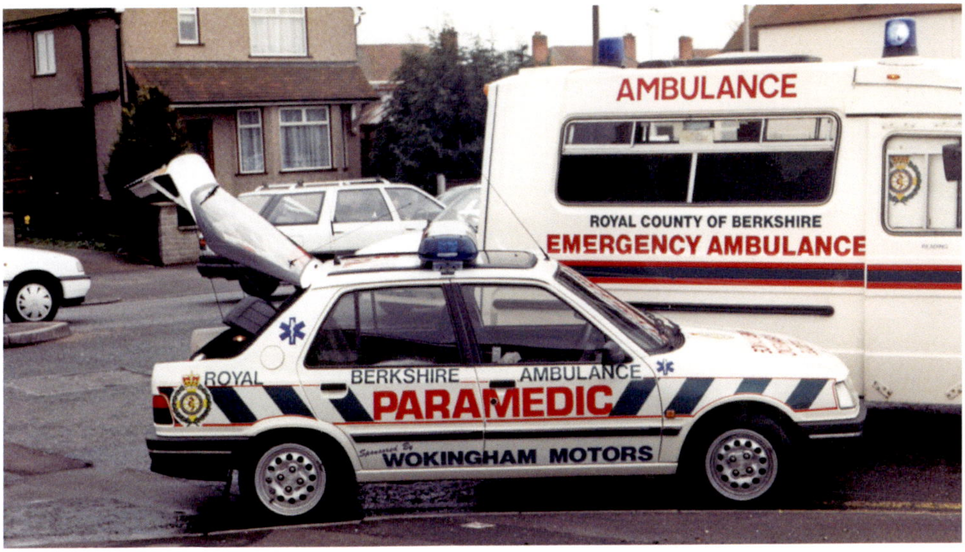

Seen attending a RTC in the Whitley area of Reading during the early 1990s is another of the RBAS's varied fleet of RRVs. Call-sign Papa Mike Two, this Peugeot 309 hatchback was based at Bracknell. At the time, the RRVs were sponsored by local car dealerships. Other cars used were a Peugeot 405 saloon, a Ford Mondeo hatchback, a Saab 9-5 saloon, a VW Passat estate and a Vauxhall Vectra saloon. (Photo: Ivan Barefield)

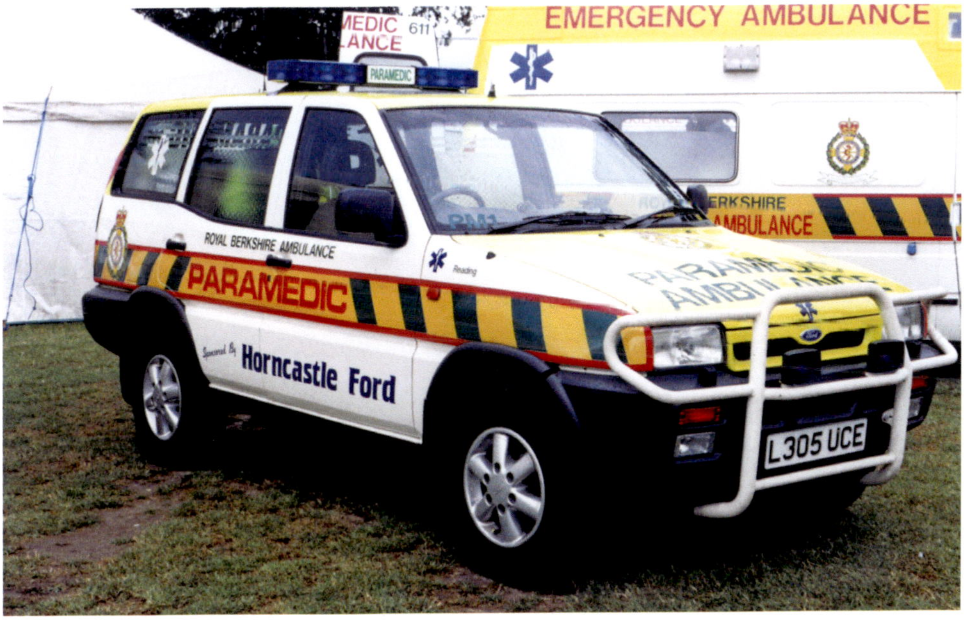

The car-based RRVs were replaced by Ford Maverick LWB 4x4s stationed at Bracknell, Maidenhead, Newbury and Reading. On display at the Berkshire Emergency Services' Tournament in Reading in 1995 was L305 UCE (1993), call-sign Papa Mike One, based at Reading and nicknamed Lucy due to the letters in its registration. The bull-bar was removed during its service due to safety concerns regarding injuries caused to pedestrians during collisions with 4x4s fitted with bull-bars.

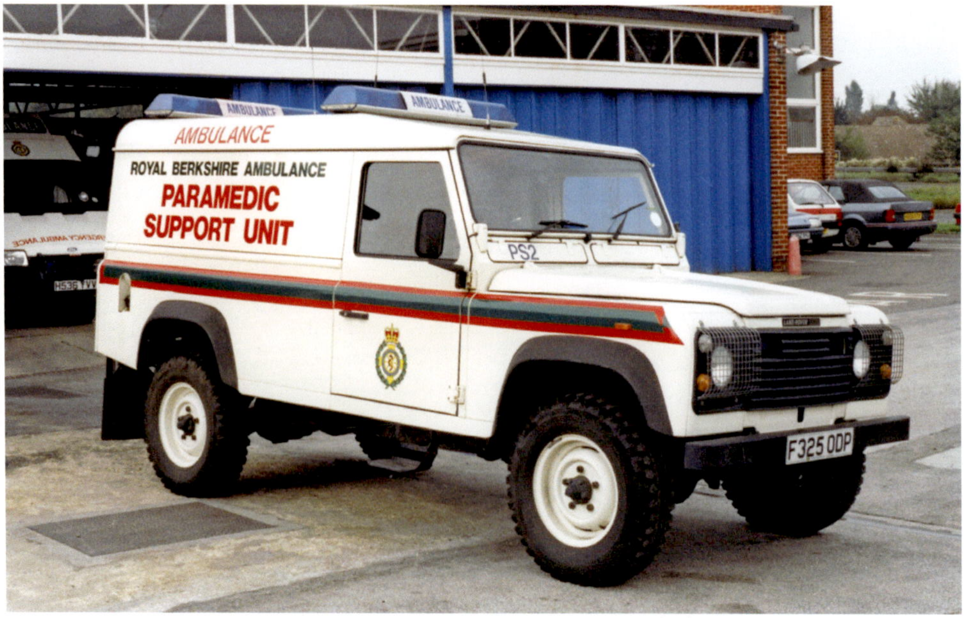

RBAS had a pair of Land Rover 110 4x4 Paramedic Support Units, which carried extra equipment to support Emergency Ambulance crews attending large incidents. F325 ODP (1988), call-sign Papa Sierra Two, was based at Newbury and primarily covered the western part of Berkshire, although both PSUs attended the large fire which engulfed part of Windsor Castle in November 1992.

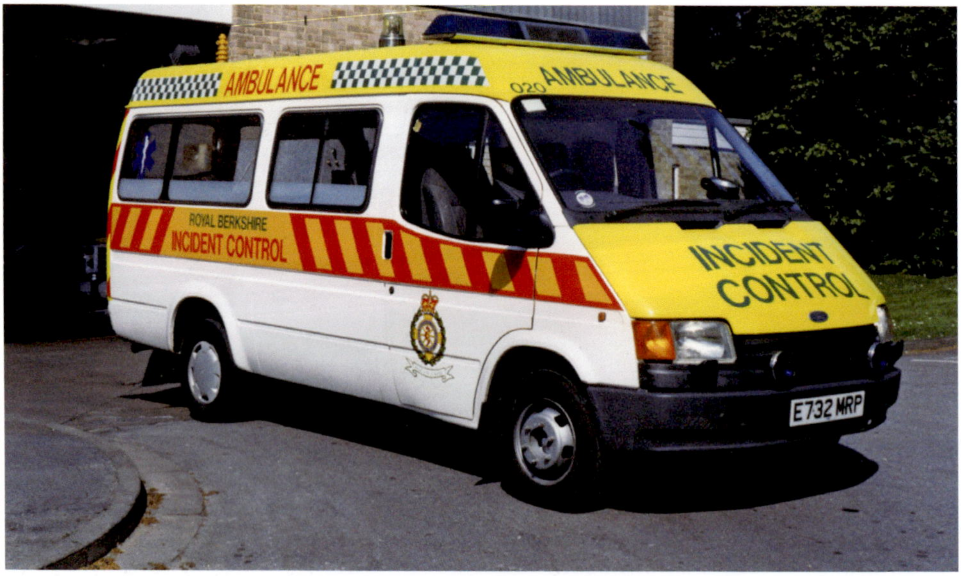

This 1988-built Ford Transit (call-sign Zero Two Zero), an ICU seen at Bracknell Ambulance Station, had been refurbished and the livery updated to a yellow front with red and orange diagonal stripes (previously green and white cheques). In 2002, RBAS repainted one of its emergency ambulances, based at Slough, from white to Euro yellow as part of a trial. The livery is now used on ambulances in England, Wales, Northern Ireland and in several other countries.

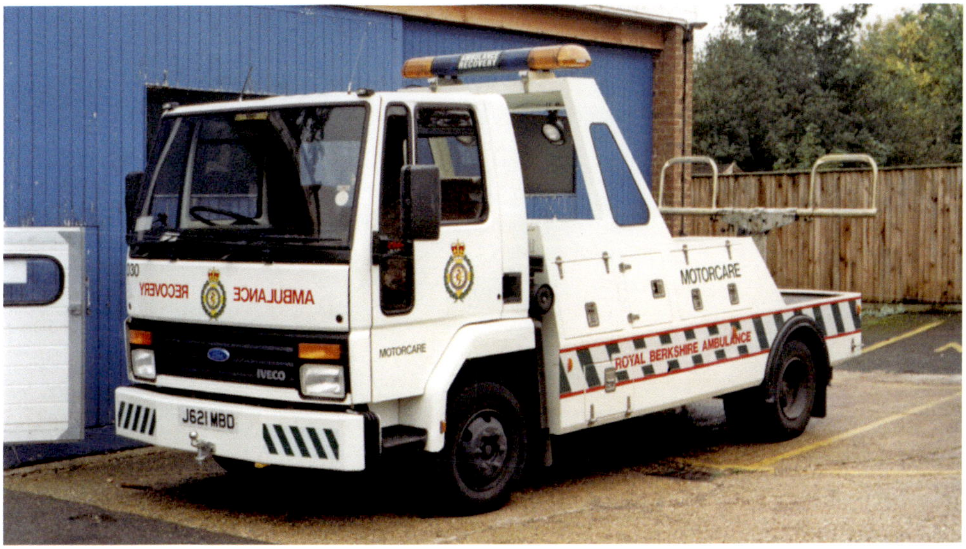

The chassis and cab of this Iveco Ford Cargo recovery vehicle were built locally at the former Iveco Ford truck plant at Langley, to the east of Slough. J621 MBD (1991/2), call-sign Zero Three Zero, was photographed outside the former Slough Ambulance Station (which was located behind Slough Fire Station), before being replaced by the new Wexham Park Ambulance Station (located within the grounds of Wexham Park Hospital).

COMMUNITY FIRST RESPONDER/F&RS CO-RESPONDER

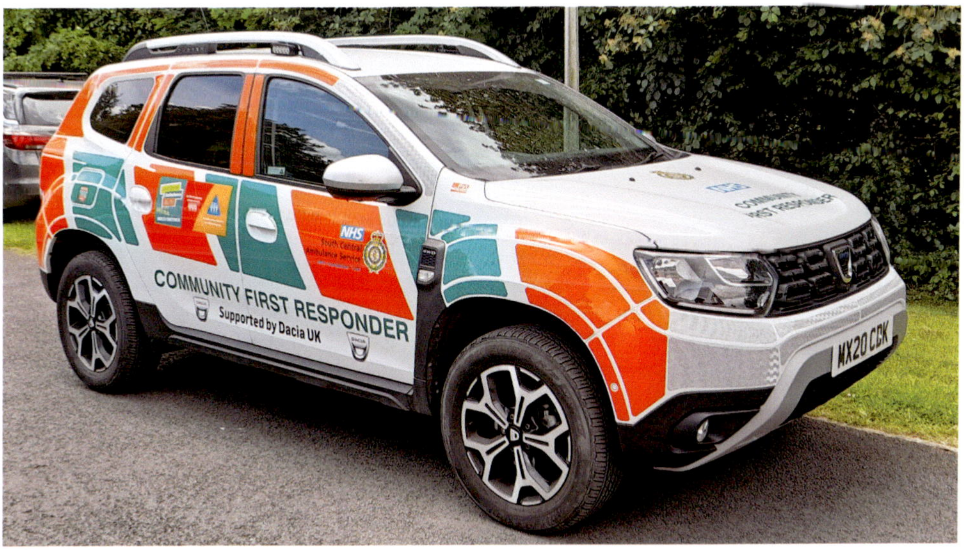

Funded by the South Central Ambulance Charity, forty Dacia Duster SUVs, known as Dynamic Response Vehicles, are available to volunteer Community First Responders (CFR) who attend certain medical emergencies in their locality. CFRs are trained in basic airway management, oxygen therapy, cardiopulmonary resuscitation and the use of automatic external defibrillators. MX20 CDK (2020) was seen at an open day at Goring Fire Station (Oxfordshire) in 2022. Of the forty Duster DRVs, twenty-seven are 4x2 versions and thirteen are 4x4s.

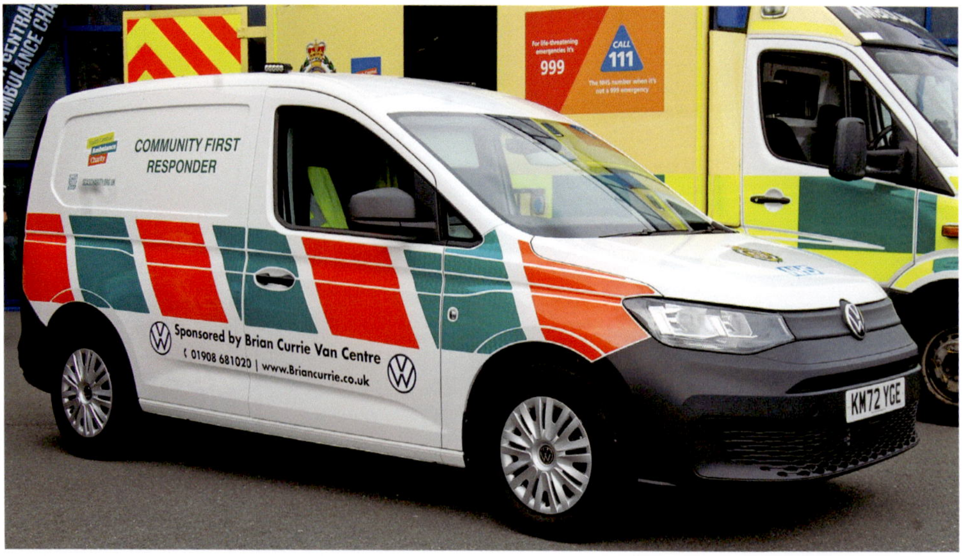

Seen at the 2024 open day at the West Ashland Blue Light Hub in Milton Keynes was this 2023 VW Caddy van, sponsored by a VW van dealer in the city. Before the bulk purchase of the Dacia Dusters in 2020, the fleet of CFR vehicles included a Ford Kuga covering Mortimer and Burghfield (Berkshire), a Land Rover Freelander covering Shinfield and Whitley (Berkshire), a Vauxhall Mokka in Didcot (Oxfordshire) and a Vauxhall Antara in Sonning Common (Oxfordshire). (Photo: Gwenifer Roberts)

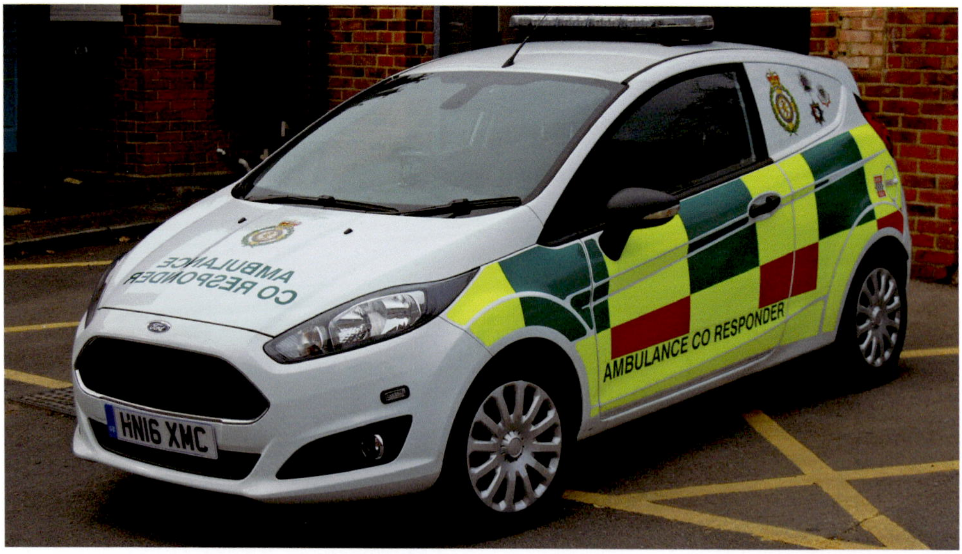

Here we see HN16 XMC (2016), a Ford Fiesta 1.5-litre diesel van used as a Co-Responder vehicle at the former Wargrave Fire Station in Berkshire. Unlike the Community Responder vehicles, the F&RS Co-Responder vehicles in the Thames Valley have blue lights, yellow, green and red Battenberg markings and most display the SCAS, Royal Berkshire, Buckinghamshire and Oxfordshire F&RS badges. Just before this photo was taken, in February 2017, the station's Dennis Sabre pump ladder had turned out to a RTC (persons trapped) on the nearby A4. Wargrave Fire Station closed in 2020.

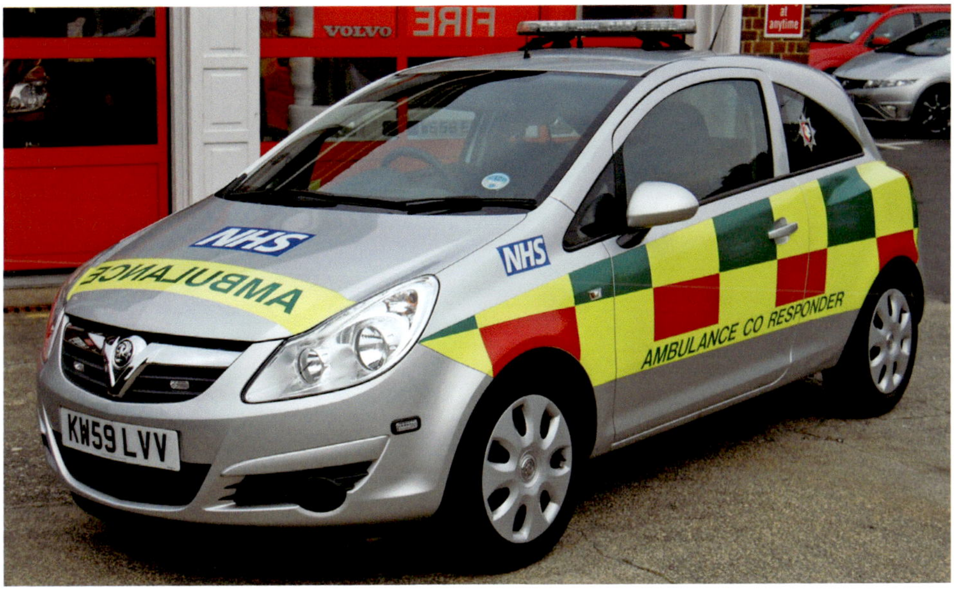

In September 2012, Great Missenden (On-Call) Fire Station in Buckinghamshire operated two fire appliances (a WrL and an OSU) and this Co-Responder vehicle: KW59 LVV (2010), a Vauxhall Corsa 1.2-litre diesel hatchback. There was at least one other Vauxhall Corsa Co-Responder vehicle in use with the Oxfordshire F&RS and two Ford Fiesta Co-Responder vehicles with the Royal Berkshire F&RS at Lambourn and Wargrave; in addition, Mortimer previously operated Ford Mondeo and Peugeot 405 CFR cars.

ROYAL AIR FORCE

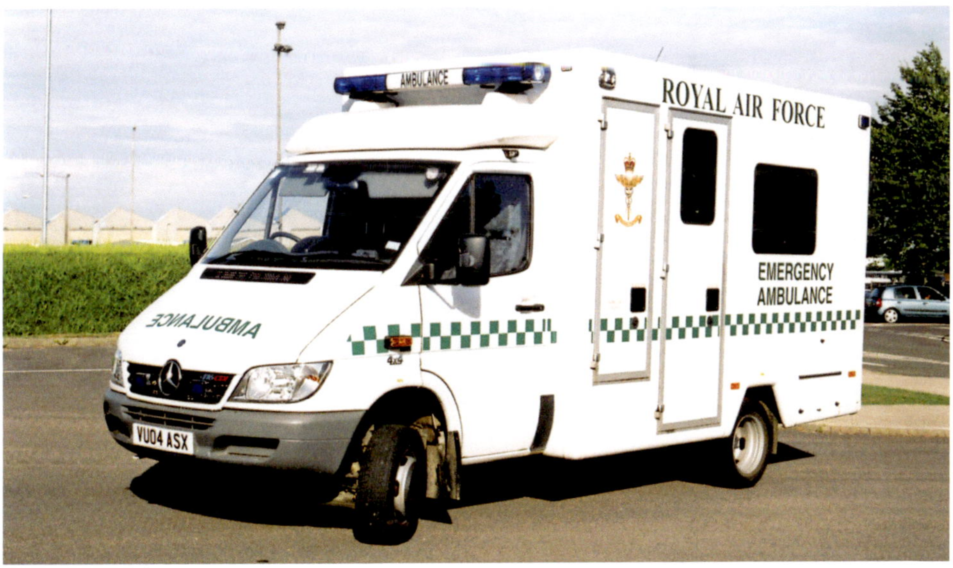

Seen while in service at RAF Brize Norton in Oxfordshire in 2006, VU04 ASX (2004) is a Mercedes Sprinter 416 CDi 4x4 Emergency Ambulance of the Royal Air Force Medical Services Branch.

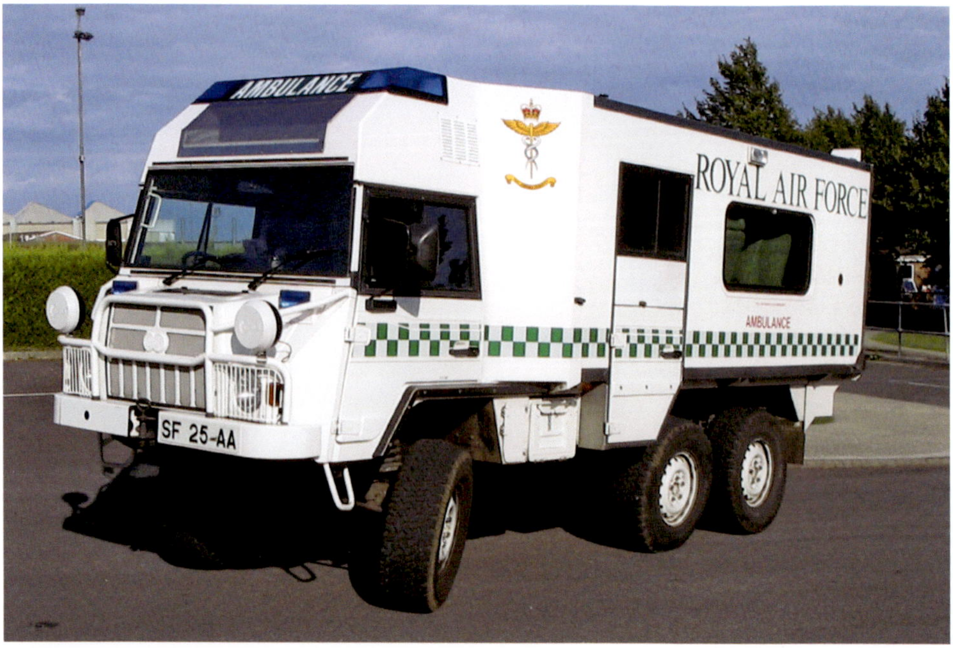

An Airfield Trauma Management Vehicle ('crash' ambulance), seen at RAF Brize Norton in 2006. Originally developed and built as 4x4 and 6x6 versions by Steyr-Daimler-Puch in Austria from the early 1970s to the late 1990s, production of the Pinzgauer was taken over by Automotive Technik in the UK in the early 2000s, with production ending in the late 2000s.

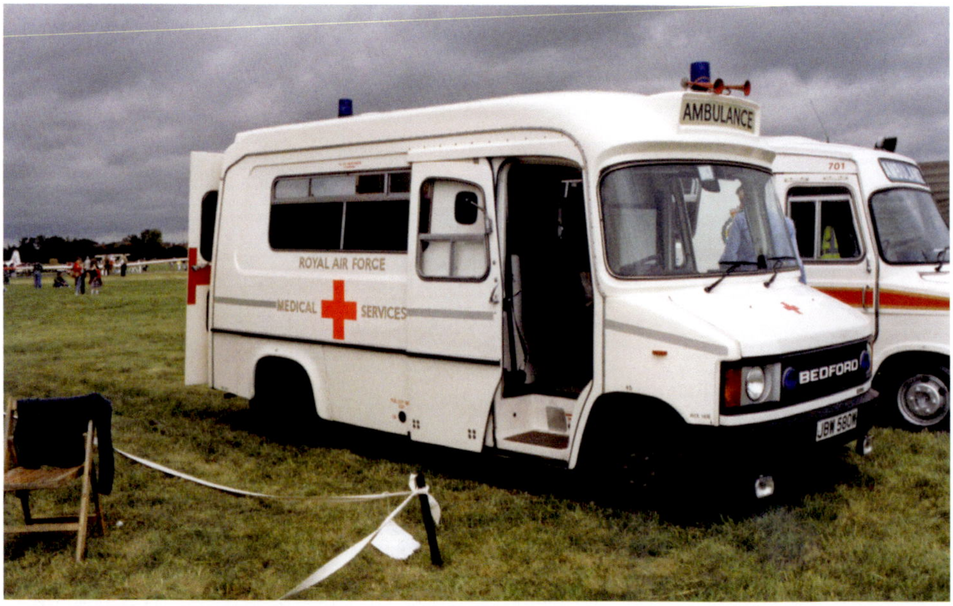

One of the ambulances providing medical cover at the Families' Day at RAF Benson in Oxfordshire in 1988 was this Bedford CF 350, bodied by Wadham Stringer. Dating from around 1981, these ambulances were supplied to both the Royal Air Force and the Army Medical Services.

In addition to the Community Responder and Fire & Rescue Service Co-Responder vehicles already featured, here is an example of a military Co-Responder vehicle. LJ14 AKG (2014), a BMW X5 4x4, was crewed by volunteer Royal Air Force personnel at RAF Benson. It was photographed when brand new at an armed forces event in Wallingford in 2014.

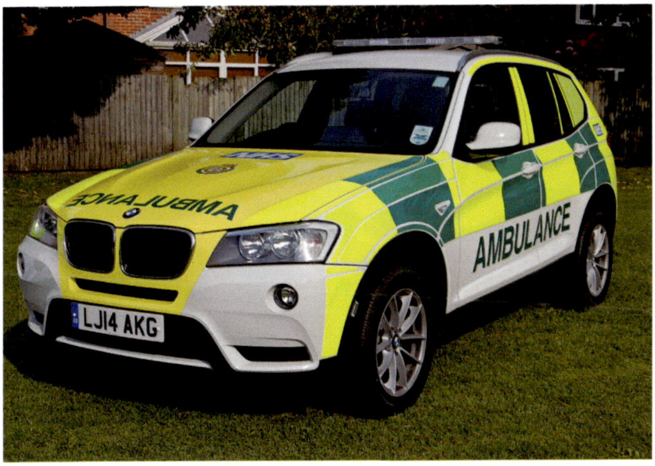

In June 1993, the Thames Valley Police held an open day at their then new Traffic Base and Vehicle Workshops in Bicester, Oxfordshire. A visitor from the United States Air Force at RAF Upper Heyford was this eighth generation Ford F350 4x4/ Wheeled Coach ambulance. In addition to the International Committee of the Red Cross and Red Crescent Societies, the Geneva Conventions allow the use of the Red Cross emblem by armed forces under strict conditions.

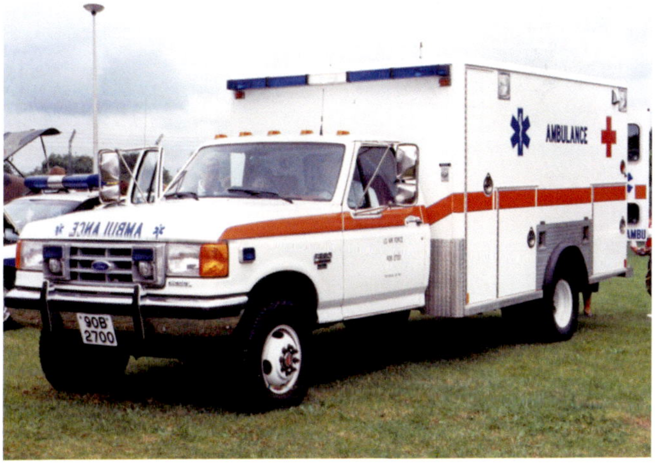

83 B 6283 (1983), a Chevrolet Custom Deluxe 30/Southern Ambulance Builders vehicle, was one of three USAF ambulances based at RAF Greenham Common in Berkshire in 1988. Greenham Common became well known as the main UK base for US cruise missiles carrying nuclear warheads, the other base being RAF Molesworth in Cambridgeshire. Greenham Common was the scene of many protests in the 1980s. Although the base closed in 1992, a peace camp remained until 2000.

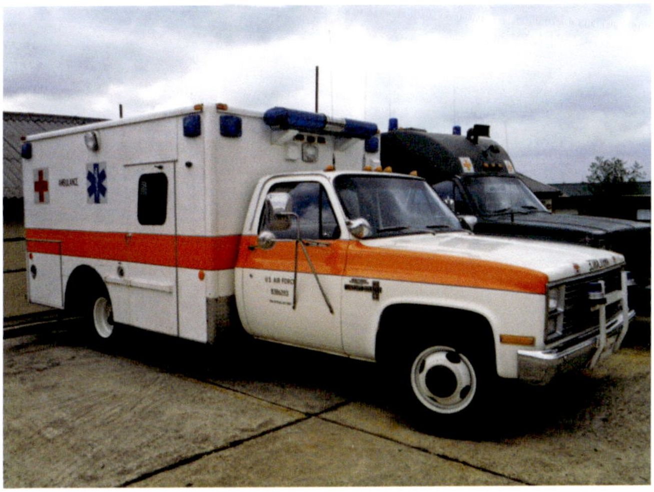

Chapter 2
Fire & Rescue Services

The Thames Valley is covered by three local authority fire and rescue services (F&RS): Buckinghamshire, Oxfordshire and Royal Berkshire, with a joint Thames Valley Fire Control located at Calcot in West Berkshire and a back-up facility at Kidlington in Oxfordshire. A number of military, aviation and industrial sites have their own fire cover.

Buckinghamshire F&RS has nineteen fire stations (five whole-time/on-call, four day-crewed/on-call and ten on-call), covering an area of 1,874 square kilometres (724 square miles), with headquarters, workshops and an Urban Search and Rescue Team in Aylesbury, and a training facility at Haddenham. With a population of over 800,000, the largest urban areas are the new city of Milton Keynes, the county town of Aylesbury and High Wycombe. Major risks include the world-renowned Pinewood Film Studios, the historic Bletchley Park, the rail maintenance centre at Wolverton, and His Majesty's Government Communications Centre at Hanslope Park. The main transport routes include the M1, M4, M25 and M40 motorways, the A41 trunk road, the West Coast Main Line and the Chiltern Main Line (the HS2 high-speed railway line is currently under construction through the south of Buckinghamshire).

Oxfordshire F&RS has twenty-five fire stations (three whole-time/on-call, three day-crewed/on-call and nineteen on-call), covering an area of 2,605 square kilometres (1,006 square miles), with headquarters and workshops in Kidlington, and a training facility at Didcot. With a population of over 691,000, the largest urban areas are the university city of Oxford, Banbury and Bicester. Major risks include the UNESCO World Heritage Site of Blenheim Palace, the science research centres at Culham and Harwell, Oxford Airport and RAF Brize Norton. The main transport routes include the M40 motorway, the A34 and A40 trunk roads, the Great Western Main Line, the Cherwell Valley Line and the Chiltern Main Line (the HS2 high-speed railway line is currently under construction through the north of Oxfordshire).

Royal Berkshire F&RS has sixteen fire stations (eleven whole-time, one whole-time/on-call and four on-call), covering an area of 1,263 square kilometres (488 square miles), with headquarters at Calcot and a small maintenance facility at Theale Fire Station (major servicing and vehicle maintenance is carried out under a contract with the Hampshire and Isle of Wight F&RS at their workshops in Eastleigh), and a training facility at Whitley Wood. With a population of over 911,000, the largest urban areas are the county town of Reading, the industrial town of Slough and the new town of Bracknell. Major risks include Slough Industrial Estate, the Atomic Weapons Establishments at Aldermaston and Burghfield, and the world-famous, historic Windsor Castle. The main transport routes include the M4, M25, A308(M) (the shortest motorway in England), A329(M) and A404(M) motorways, the A4 and A34 trunk roads, the Great Western Main Line and the Reading–Taunton Line.

BUCKINGHAMSHIRE

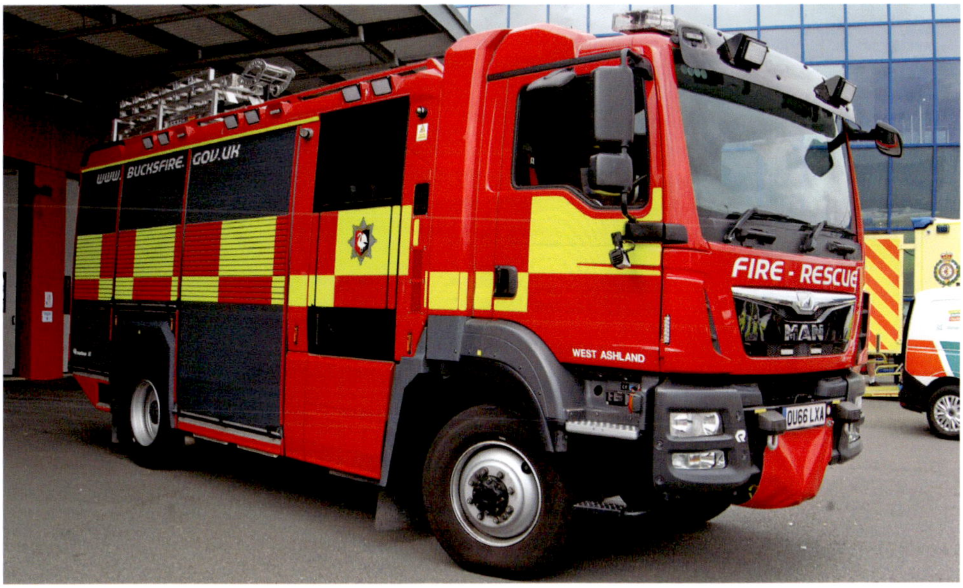

In 2016, three continental-style, all-wheel-drive water tenders were bought to replace three water tenders bodied by Emergency One on Mercedes Unimog 4x4 chassis. Built on MAN TGM 4x4 chassis, they feature Rosenbauer AT (Aluminium Technology) bodywork. The three appliances were allocated to Aylesbury, High Wycombe and Great Holm (now at West Ashland). Call-sign One Six Papa Three was seen at the third annual open day at the West Ashland Blue Light Hub in August 2024.

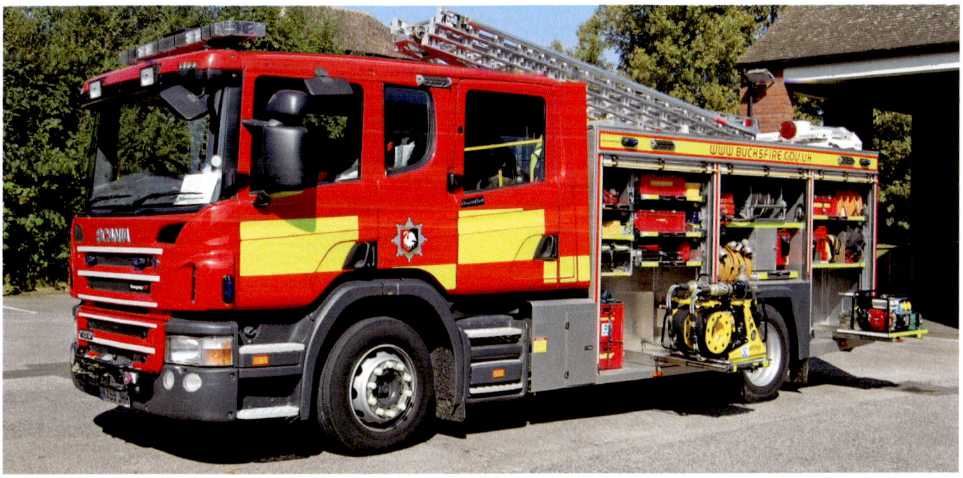

Having had one of the most varied fleets in the country between the late 1980s and mid-2000s, standardisation of pumping appliances started in 2005 with the introduction of Scania P series chassis bodied by Emergency One. On the run at the day-crewed station at Buckingham in 2012 was KX59 JHH (2009), a Scania P270. Since 2017, Emergency One has built Thames Valley specification pumping appliances, on Volvo FLH chassis, for Buckinghamshire, purchased with Oxfordshire and Royal Berkshire.

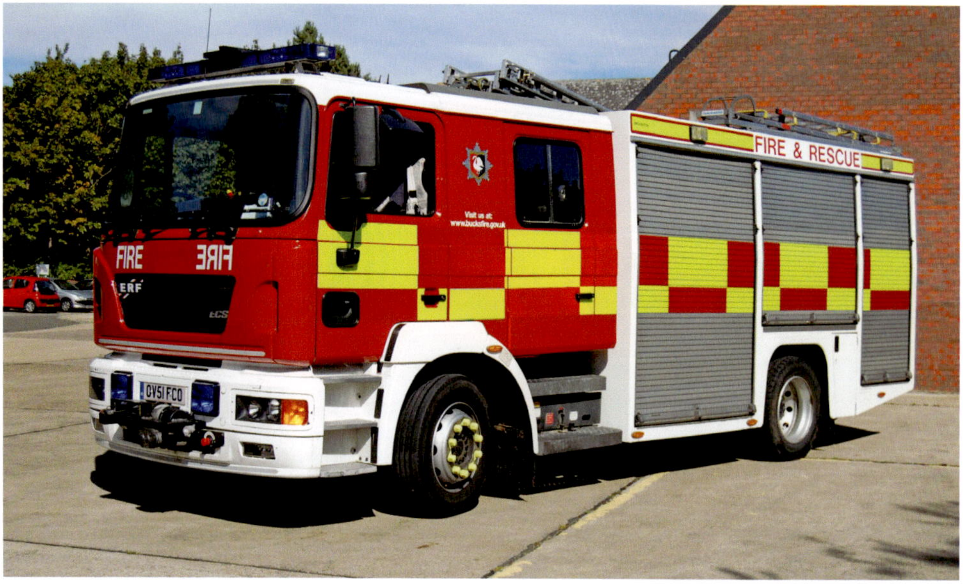

During the late 1960s and throughout the 1970s, ERF chassis were used as the basis for pumping appliances, aerial appliances and special appliances, before a very quiet period during the 1980s. ERF chassis began being used for fire appliances again in the late 1980s. Some of the last ERF appliances were built for Buckinghamshire. On the run at Broughton Fire Station in Milton Keynes in 2012 was Rescue Pump, OV51 FCO (2001), built by TVAC on an ERF ECS chassis.

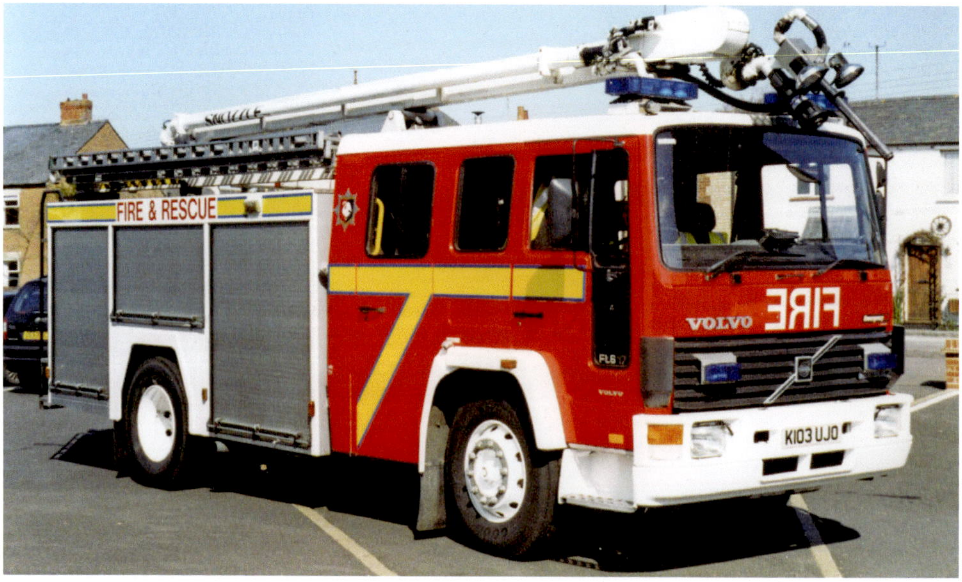

K103 UJO (1992), a Volvo FL6.17 chassis, was originally bodied as a water carrier, based at Princes Risborough. It was later rebuilt by Emergency One and fitted with a 15-metre (50-foot) Snozzle boom by GB Fire, serving at Aylesbury and then Waddesdon. Reminiscent of the Simonitor appliances (used in Clwyd, Durham, Essex, Hampshire, Lancashire, Greater Manchester and West Yorkshire in the 1970s), it can be compared with today's Stingers in Lancashire and Scorpions in Cheshire and Greater Manchester.

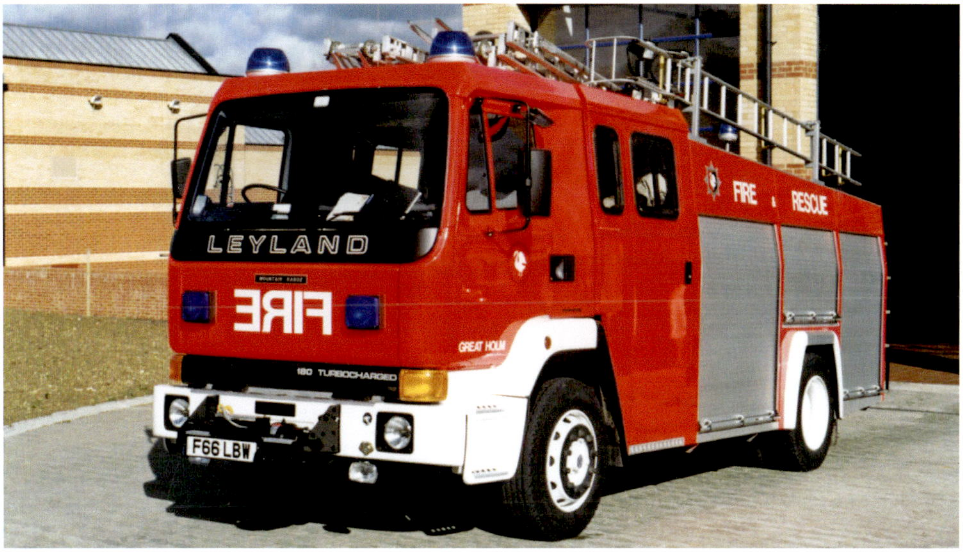

A new chassis manufacturer was added to Buckinghamshire's then mainly Dodge-based fleet in 1989, when two RPs were delivered in a new fluorescent orange/red and white livery. Built on Leyland Freighter 17.18 chassis by Mountain Range, they were powered by 6.5-litre, 180-hp, turbocharged diesel engines. F66 LBW was photographed outside the then brand-new Great Holm Fire Station in the west of Milton Keynes, which, along with Bletchley Fire Station, has been replaced by a new, tri-service blue light hub at West Ashland. (Photo: Colin Dunford)

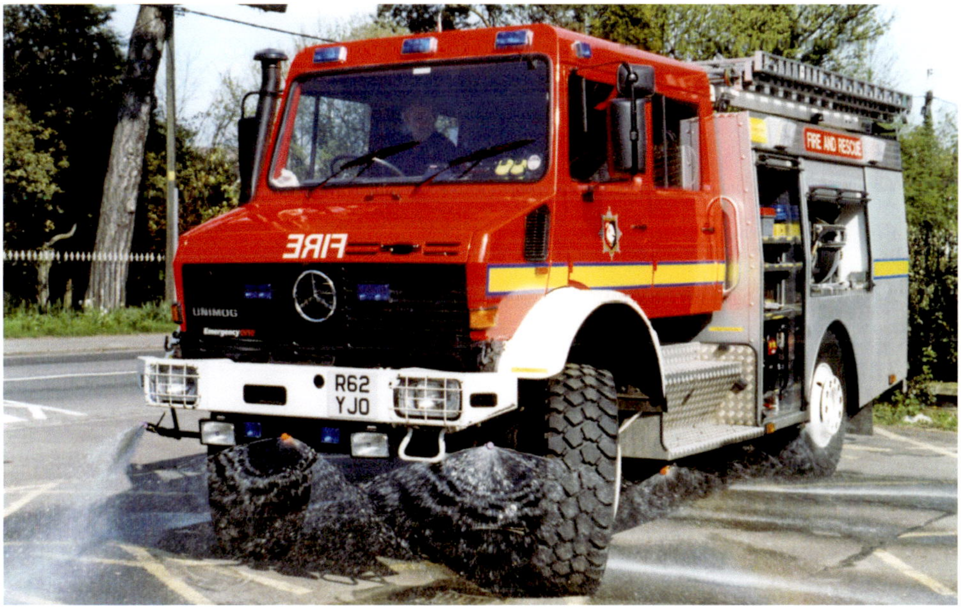

Before being replaced by the MAN 4x4 pumps, Buckinghamshire operated three other continental-style, all-wheel-drive light water tenders. Seen here at Stokenchurch, demonstrating its water spray system, is R62 YJO, one of two Mercedes Unimog 4x4 chassis bodied by Emergency One in 1997; a third identical appliance arrived in 2000. They served at various stations within the county including Aylesbury, Great Holm and High Wycombe.

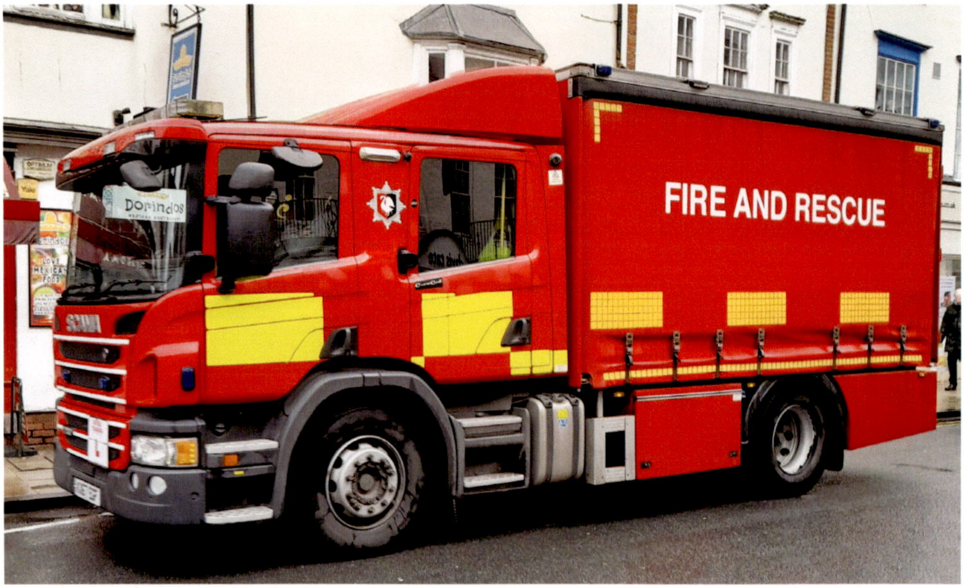

A frequent visitor to Oxfordshire is Buckinghamshire's Driver Training Vehicle KX67 EGF (2017), a Scania P280 fitted with a factory-built CP28 crew cab with air deflector and curtain-side body by Bence. It was photographed moving off from standing traffic in High Street, Abingdon, after pulling out of the drill yard of Abingdon Fire Station a few minutes before. The small black circle to the right of the crew cab door is a CCTV camera, now common on many emergency vehicles.

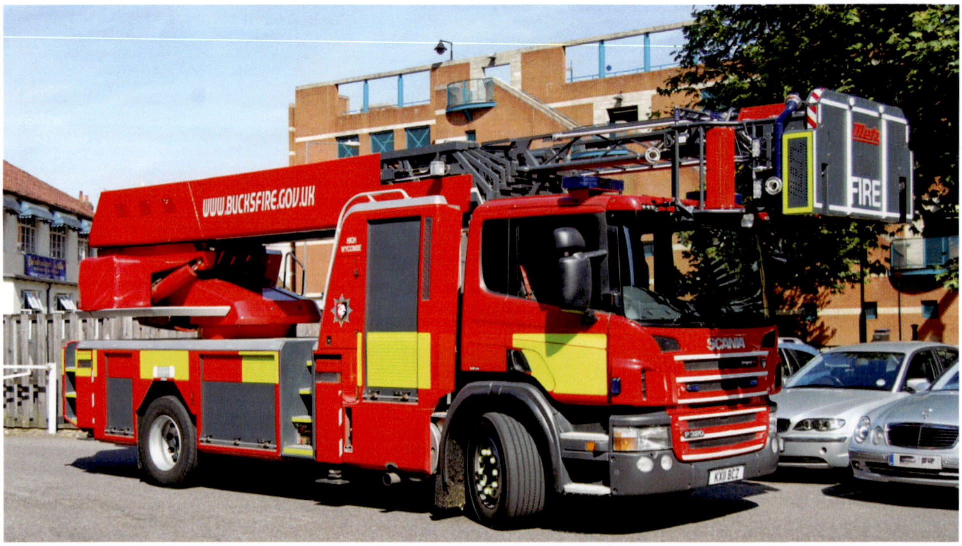

Having operated a mix of turntable ladders and hydraulic platforms of various heights as aerial appliances, a new TL was placed on the run at High Wycombe in 2011. Supplied by Emergency One, KX11 BCZ is based on a Scania P320 chassis and carries a Metz-Rosenbauer L32A-XS, five section, 32-metre (105-foot) ladder, with an articulated top section and a rescue cage with a capacity of 450 kg or four persons. In 2014, an identical TL went on the run at Great Holm before transferring to the new Blue Light Hub at West Ashland in 2020.

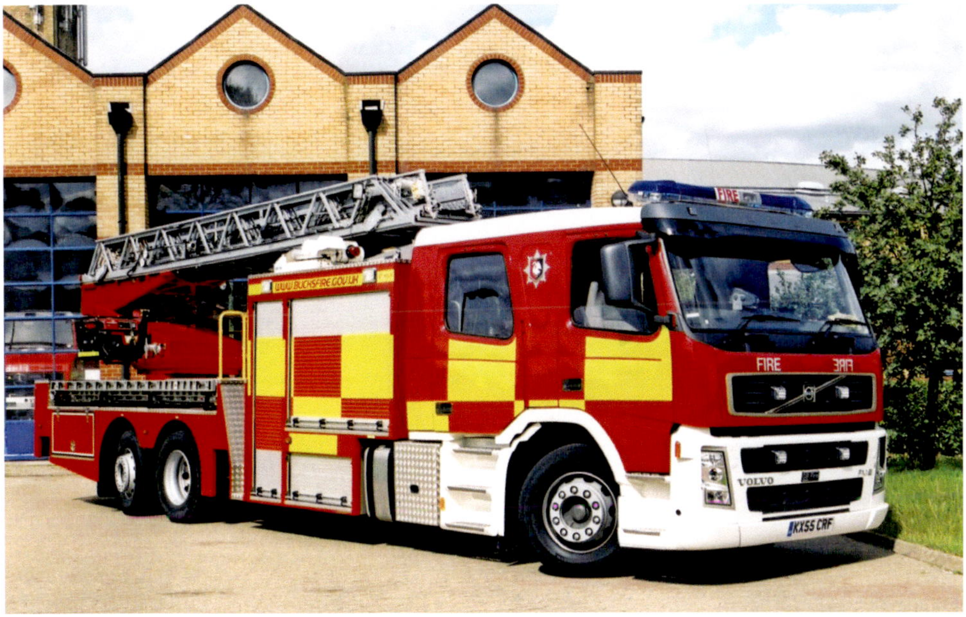

As an alternative to the aerial rescue pump appliances used in some fire and rescue services, Buckinghamshire commissioned this unique vehicle. Built by GB Fire on a three-axle Volvo FM9 chassis, it was fitted with a Magirus ladder set from an Iveco TL previously based at Newport Pagnell. KX55 CRF (2005) was based at Great Holm and operated as an aerial/water tender until it was replaced by a more conventional-style TL. (Photo: Gavin Stewart)

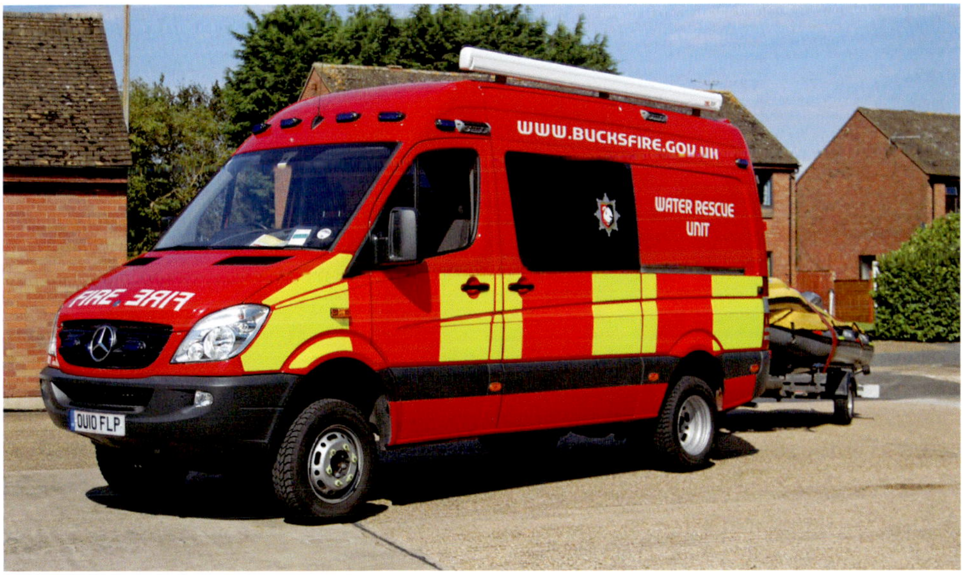

Buckinghamshire has two Water Rescue Units, based on Mercedes Sprinter 4x4 high-roof combi vans. Towing a trailer carrying an inflatable boat with outboard motor, each WRU carries water rescue personnel protective equipment, safety gear, stretchers and an inflatable rescue sledge. OU10 FLP (2010) is based at Beaconsfield in the south of the county, while OU10 FLR is based at Newport Pagnell in the north of the county.

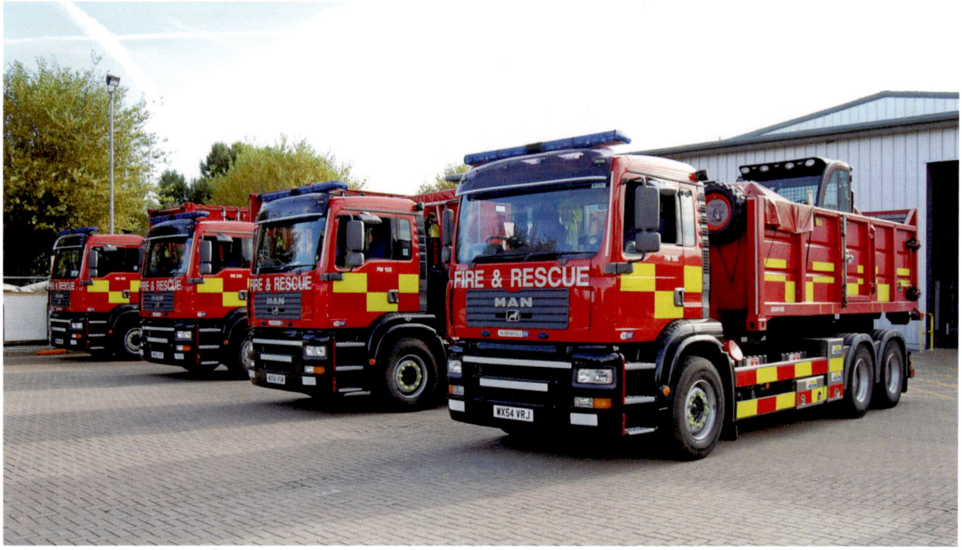

Following the terrorist attacks in the USA on 11 September 2001, twenty Urban Search and Rescue Teams were established within UK fire and rescue services under the New Dimensions programme. One of three USAR teams in the South East Region of England (along with Hampshire and Kent) is in Buckinghamshire; they were the first USAR team to attend the Didcot A Power Station collapse in 2016. Based at Aylesbury are four prime movers, five USAR modules (pods), two L4Vs and one search dog unit.

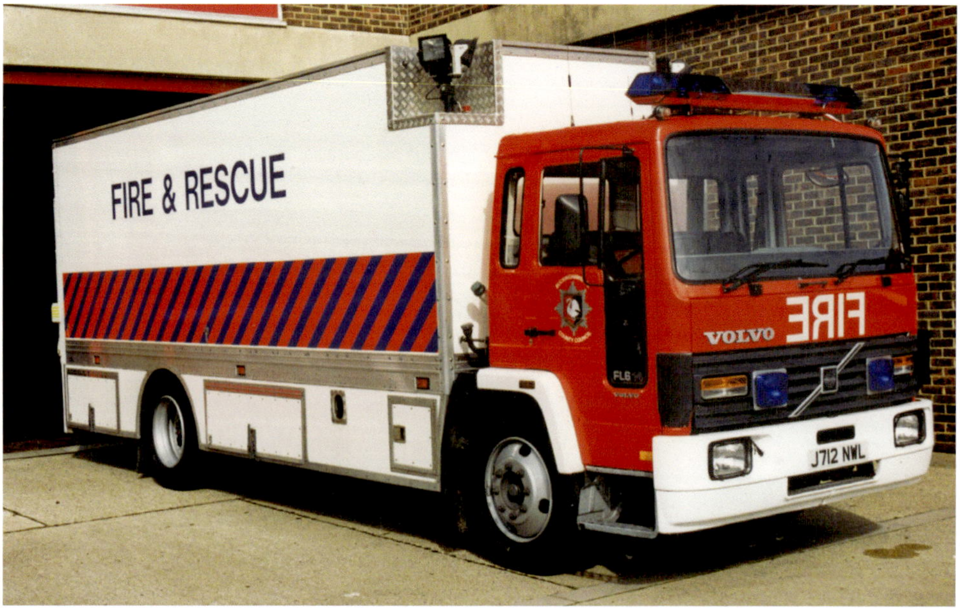

In the early 1990s, two Operational Support Units were placed in service, based on Volvo FL6.14 chassis and bodied by Hawson. Carrying a wide range of specialist equipment, they were based at various stations including Aylesbury, Bletchley, Great Holm and High Wycombe. J712 NWL (1992) served at both High Wycombe (call-sign Wycombe Six) and, as shown here, at the old Aylesbury Fire Station in Cambridge Street (call-sign Aylesbury Six). (Photo: Gavin Stewart)

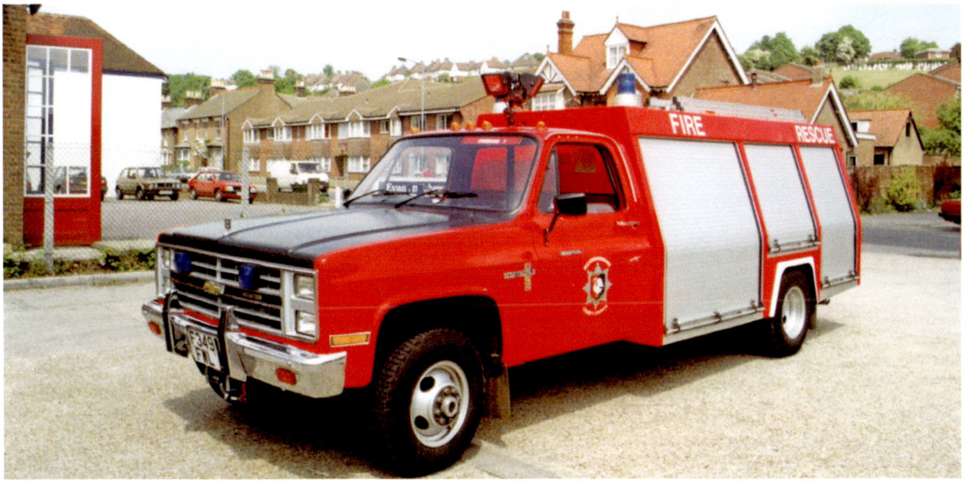

F349 FWL (1988) is a Chevrolet K30 4x4 which had three different roles. Originally built by Mountain Range as a Motorway Support Unit for rapid response to incidents on the M25 and M40 motorways from Gerrards Cross, then High Wycombe, then Chesham (call-sign Chesham Seven). It was then rebodied by Hawson as a Breathing Apparatus Support Unit and based at Waddesdon. Finally, it was rebodied as a Light Recovery Vehicle, fitted with a spectacle lift and based at Workshops at Headquarters.

OXFORDSHIRE

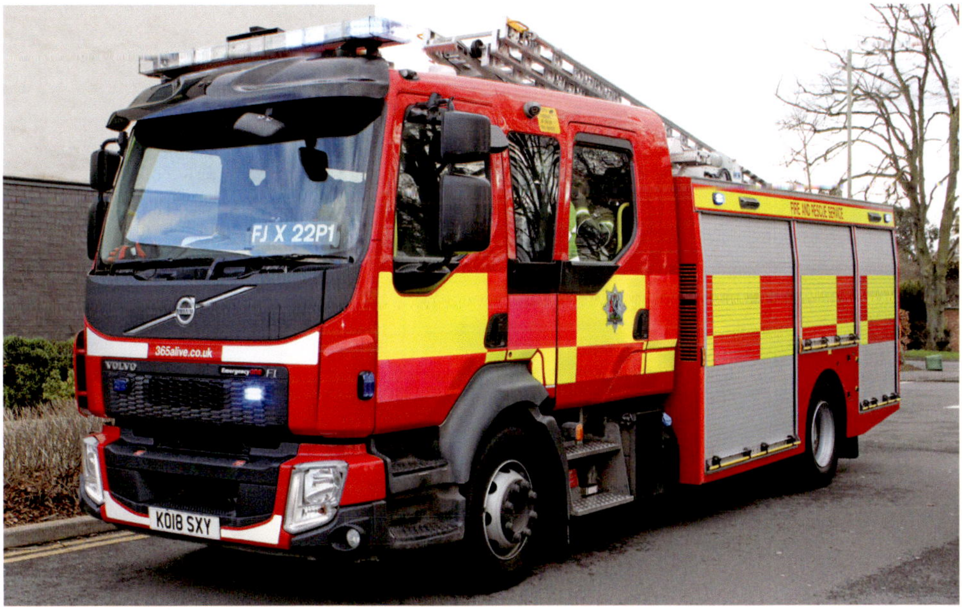

Seen attending an accidental fire alarm activation in March 2024 is Abingdon's day-crewed Water Tender Ladder (WrL) KO18 SXY (2018), one of Oxfordshire's Volvo FLH/Emergency One, Thames Valley specification pumping appliances. This appliance featured in an article on Emergency Fire Appliance Driving instruction on *Crimewatch Live* on BBC television in 2020. (Photo: Gethin Roberts)

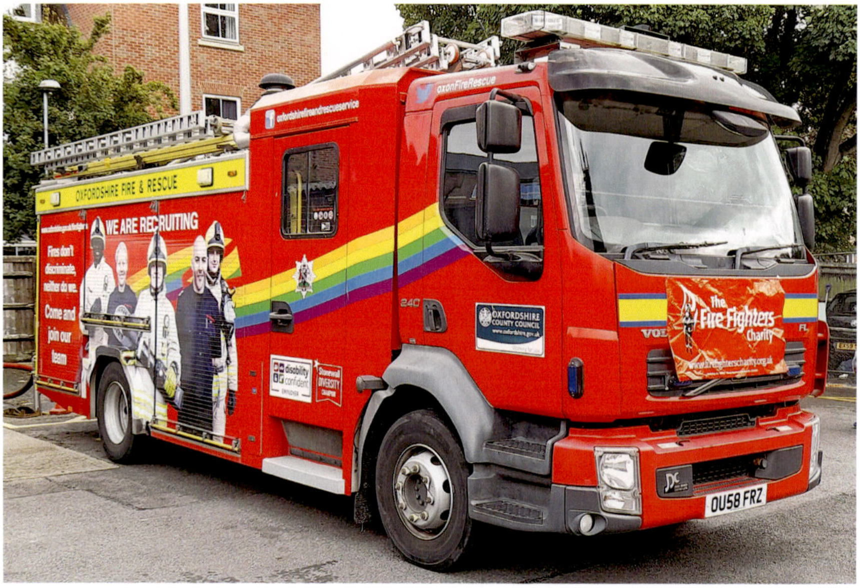

Having used Austin and Bedford chassis for pumping appliances, Oxfordshire has used Volvo chassis since the late 1980s; first the FL6.14, followed by the FLH. OU58 FRZ (2009), bodied by John Dennis Coachbuilders (JDC), often attends public events, 'have-a-go' recruitment sessions and open days promoting diversity and inclusion, such as at Abingdon in 2024, when the day-crewed station (built by the Berkshire and Reading Fire Brigade) celebrated its sixtieth anniversary.

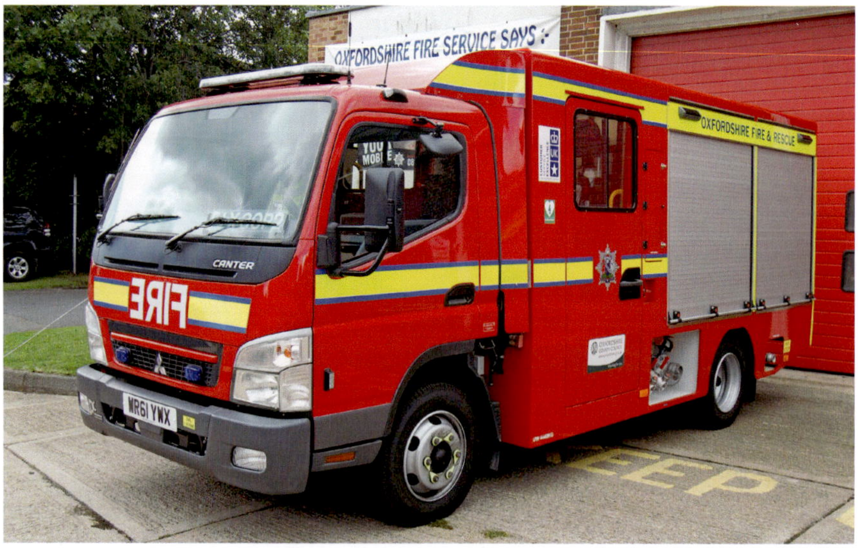

Two JDC, ex-demonstration, compact pumping appliances were purchased for trial use as second pumps at two pump stations. WR61 YWX (2012), a Mitsubishi Canter/JDC, was seen on the run as the second (on-call) pump at Slade Park in Oxford in 2015 (call-sign Three Zero Papa Two). An almost identical machine (but with yellow roller shutters), WR61 PWF (2011), was used as a Young Firefighters' appliance. Both appliances had mid-mounted pumps with the hose connections on the near side.

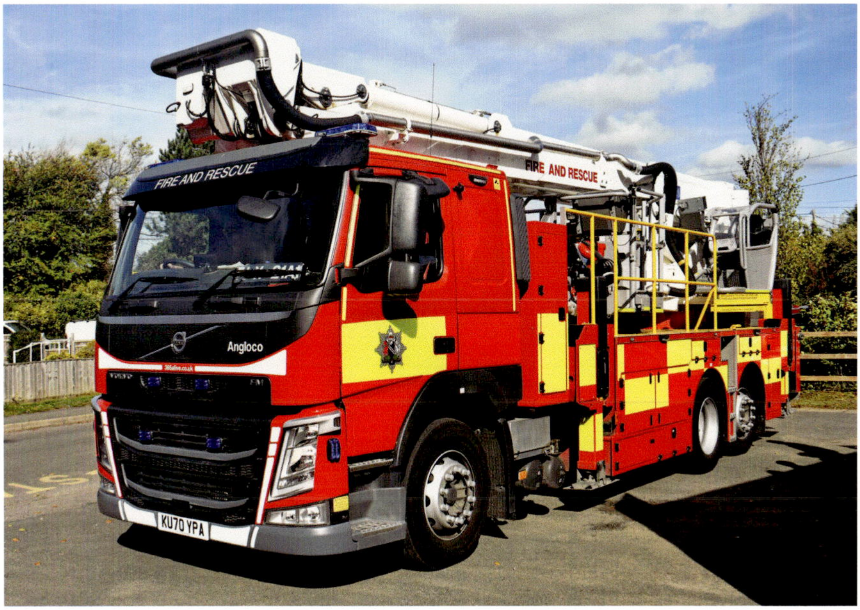

Attending the open day at Goring Fire Station in October 2022 was the hydraulic platform based at Rewley Road Fire Station in Oxford. Call-sign Two One Alpha One, KU70 YPA (2020) is a Volvo FM/Angloco/Bronto. Previously, Oxfordshire operated two different Volvo aerial ladder platforms and an ERF hydraulic platform.

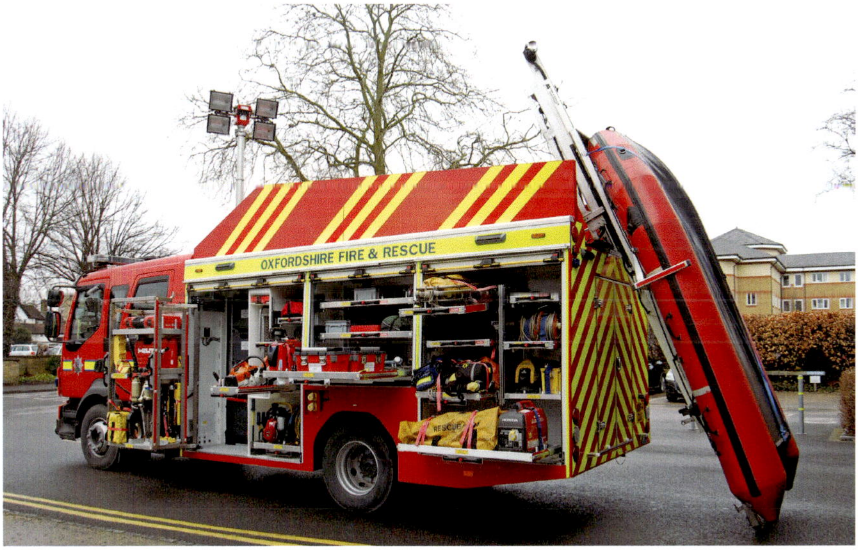

Photographed after returning from a pile-up on the M40 involving around thirty-five vehicles, at which the crew extricated one casualty, was Oxfordshire's very comprehensively equipped Volvo FLH/JDC, Rescue Tender, OU64 CUC (2015), call-sign Zero Six Romeo One. Equipment includes front-mounted remote-controlled winch, light-mast, roof-mounted Avon inflatable boat on a powered gantry, generator, two sets of Weber hydraulic rescue tools, LGV rescue platform, shoring equipment, numerous power and hand tools, chainsaws, animal rescue gear, water rescue gear, rope rescue gear and trauma kit.

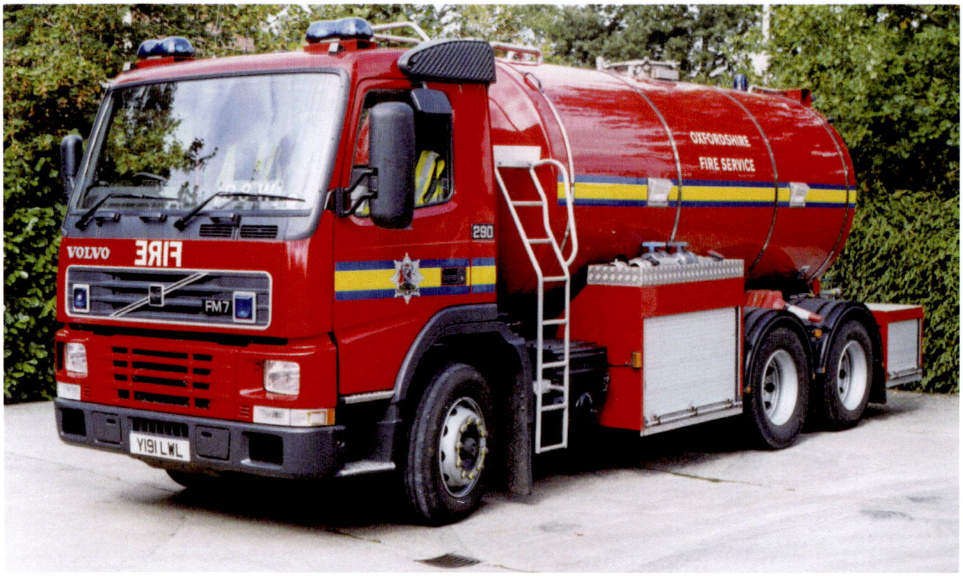

Oxfordshire has one water carrier, call-sign Two Eight Whisky One, based at Wheatley to the east of Oxford. Y191 LWL (2001) was built on a three-axle Volvo FM7 chassis. Equipment carried includes an inflatable dam and foam. Previously, Oxfordshire had two smaller water carriers, based on Volvo FL and Leyland Freighter chassis.

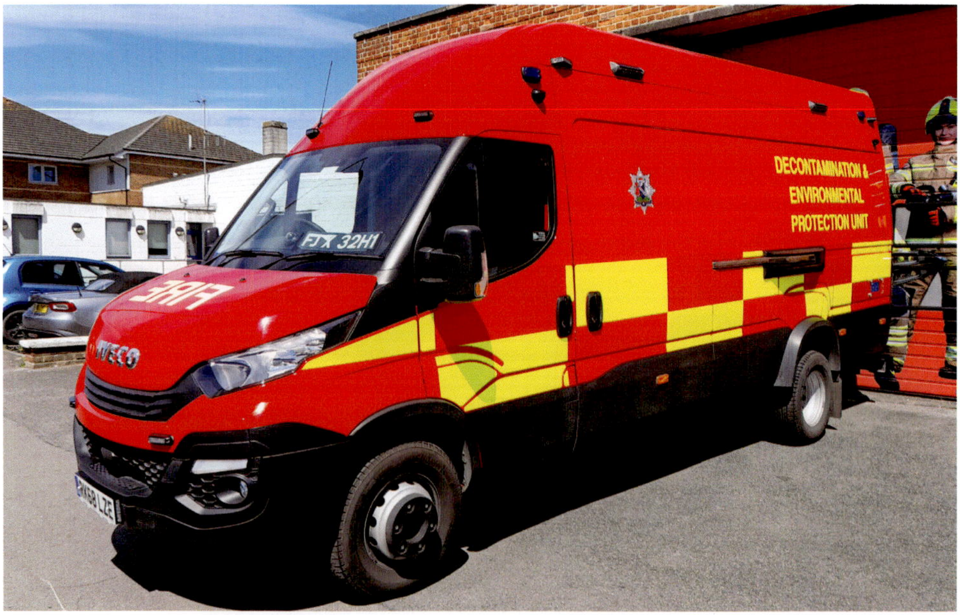

Oxfordshire's Decontamination and Environmental Protection Unit is based at Didcot in the south of the county, close to the A34, Milton Park industrial estate and the Culham and Harwell science research centres. Call-sign Three Two Hotel One, RK68 LZE (2018) is an Iveco Daily 70-180 LWB high-roof van, fitted with a Palfinger tail-lift. Equipment carried includes an inflatable dam, over drums, absorbent mats and granules, sealing putty, chemical/fuel pump and hoses, mercury spill kit, generator, gas monitors and radiation monitors. (Photo: Gethin Roberts)

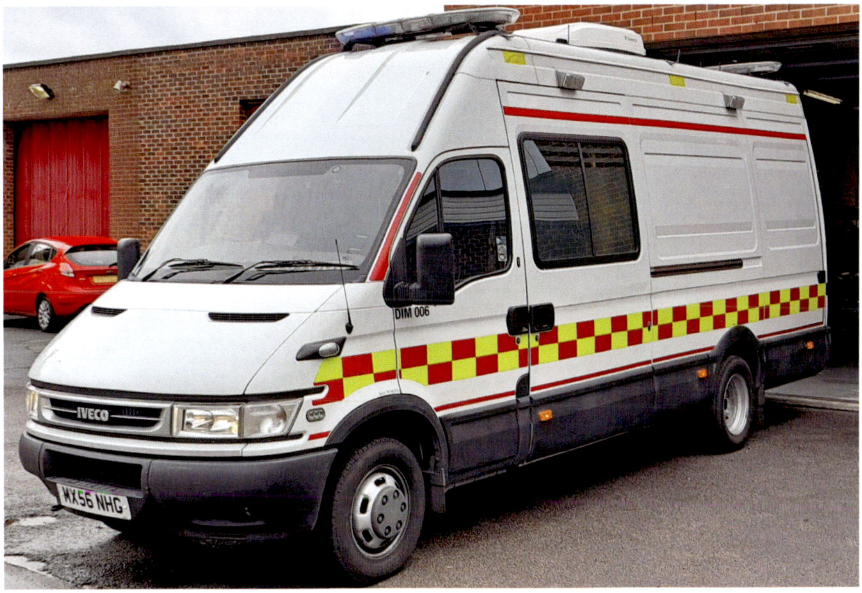

As part of the New Dimensions programme in the 2000s, twenty Detection Identification and Monitoring Units were allocated to a small number of fire and rescue services. The only DIM Unit in the Thames Valley is based at Bicester. DIM 006, MX56 NHG (2006), call-sign Zero Seven Hotel Eight, is an Iveco Daily 50C17 fitted out by AES. It carries DIM equipment to respond to incidents suspected to involve chemical, biological, radiological and nuclear materials, along with breathing apparatus, gas-tight suits, firefighter decontamination and communications equipment.

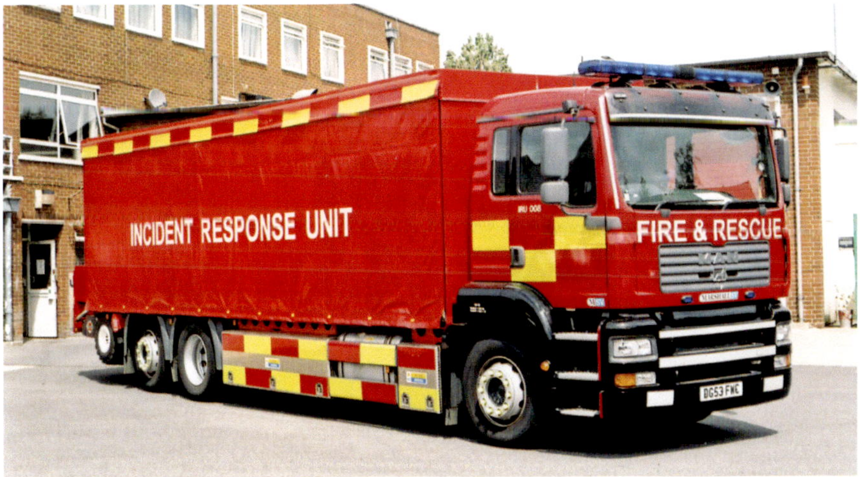

As part of the New Dimensions programme, eighty Incident Response Units were allocated to fire and rescue services. Based on MAN TGA 26.363 6x2 chassis, they were bodied by Marshall Specialist Vehicles. The IRUs carried a Moffett Mounty fork-lift truck, mass decontamination equipment, DIM equipment, gas-tight suits, re-robe packs and ancillary equipment to provide decontamination at CBRN or hazmat incidents. IRU 008, DG53 FWC (2004), call-sign Three Zero Hotel Nine, was based at Slade Park in Oxford. All IRUs have been withdrawn, with some replaced by dis-robe pods.

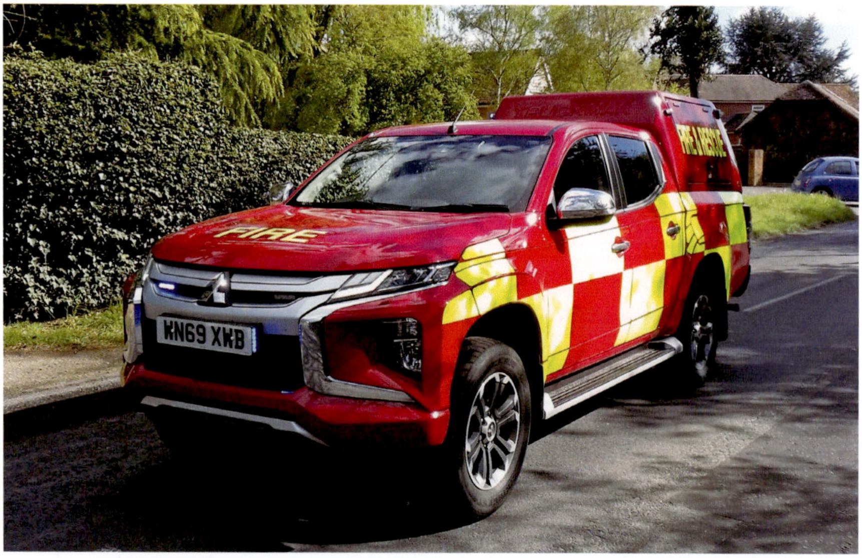

An Incident Support Officer from Witney arrives at the scene of flooding, caused by a burst water main, on Reading Road in Winterbrook, just south of Wallingford, in May 2021. This Light Four Wheel Drive Vehicle, WN69 XWB (2019), is a Mitsubishi L200 4x4, fitted with a Truckman top over the load-bed. Equipment carried includes a thermal imaging camera, gas monitors, Automatic External Defibrillator (AED), medical kit, collapsible cones, lighting, throw lines and bottled water.

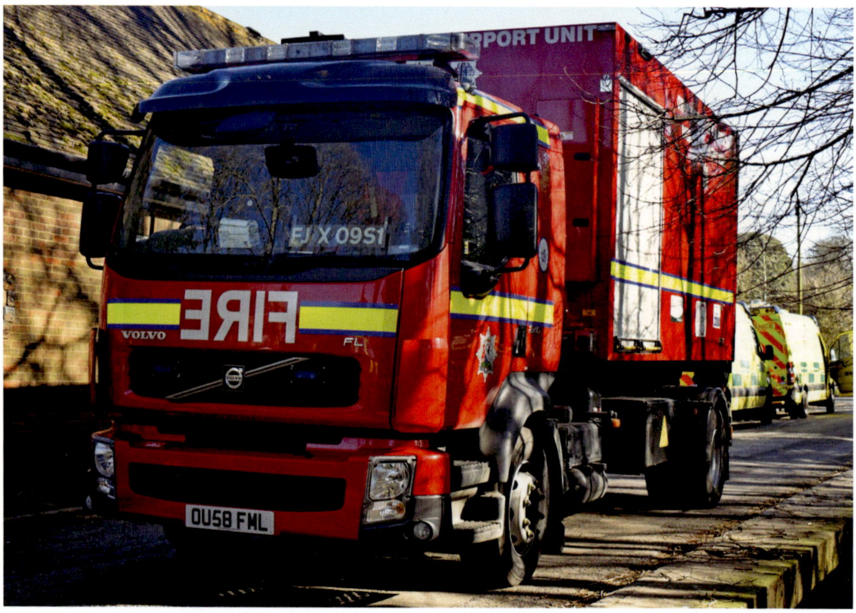

Ewelme in south Oxfordshire is a quintessential English village with a church, village hall, pub, shop, duck pond, babbling brook and houses with thatched roofs. Attending a Make Pumps Ten fire involving a thatched roof on Sunday 27 February 2022 was a Volvo FLH prime mover from Eynsham, carrying an Incident Support Unit pod built by JDC. Avoiding overhanging branches is OU58 FML (2008), call-sign Zero Nine Sierra One.

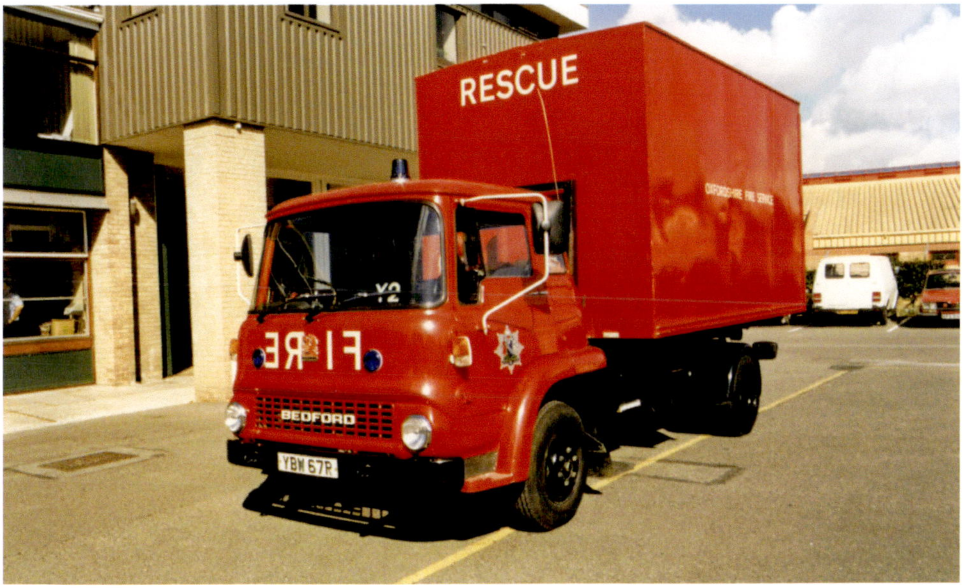

In the mid-1970s, the Oxfordshire Fire Service was one of the first to use demountable pods, standing for 'Platform on Demand'. Prior to the arrival of the purpose-built Bedford TL/HCB-Angus RT, a rescue pod was placed on the run at Kidlington. Photographed in August 1986 was YBW 67R (1976), one of three Bedford TK tractor units/chassis units in the fleet (known as prime movers elsewhere), call-sign Yankee Two; Yankee One was also based at Kidlington and Yankee Three was based at Rewley Road Fire Station in Oxford.

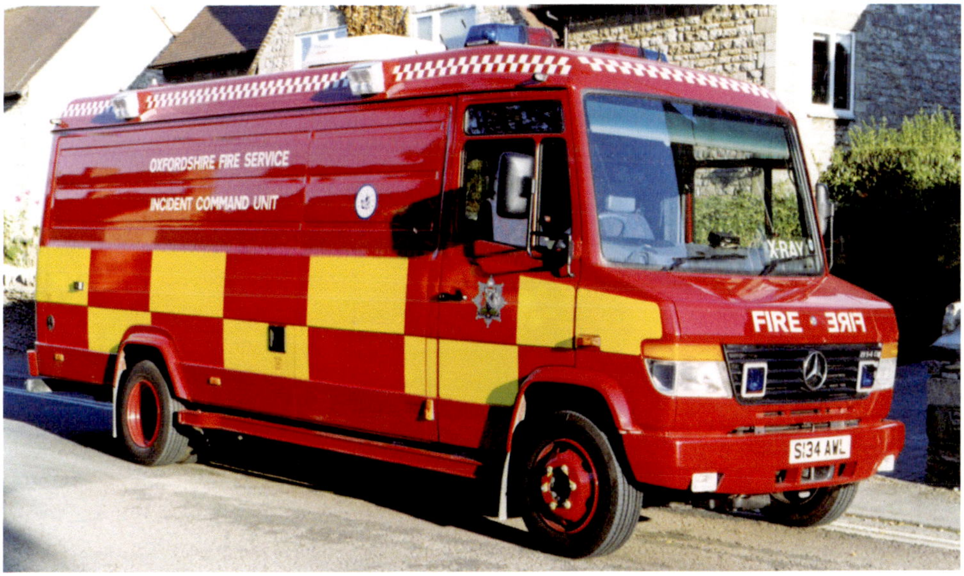

In the late 1990s, Olympic Coachbuilders in Didcot converted three Mercedes Vario 814D LWB vans into an EPU, ICU and ISU for Oxfordshire. Woodstock was initially the base for the ICU, S134 AWL (1998), call-sign X-Ray. For several years it was the only appliance in the Oxfordshire fleet to have Battenberg markings. It is now stationed at Slade Park in Oxford, the call-sign having been changed to Three Zero Charlie One.

ROYAL BERKSHIRE

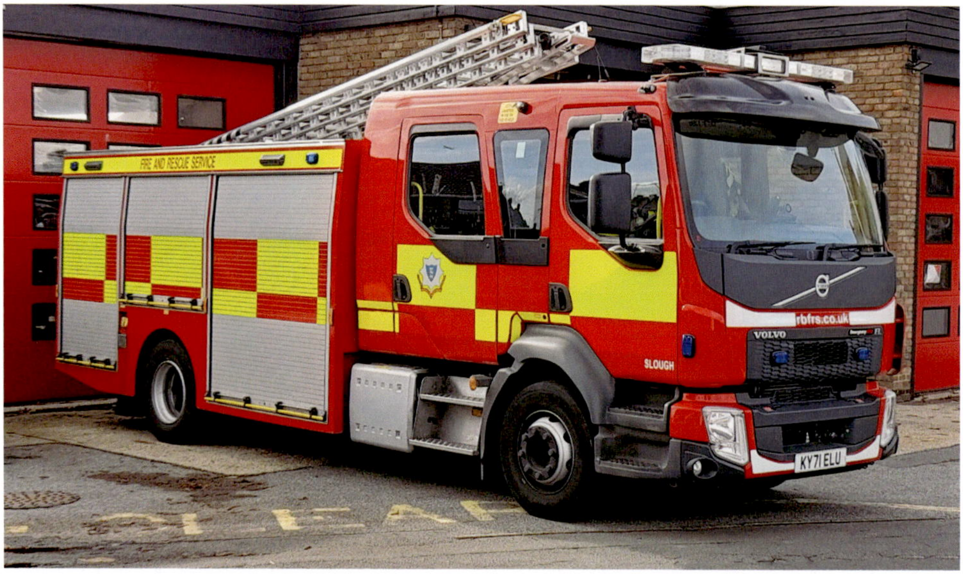

Thames Valley specification pumps were first delivered in 2017. Seen on stand-by at Langley Fire Station during that station's open day in October 2022 was the second of the two whole-time WrLs based at nearby Slough Fire Station. KY71 ELU (2021) is a Volvo FLH chassis bodied by Emergency One of Cumnock in the west of Scotland.

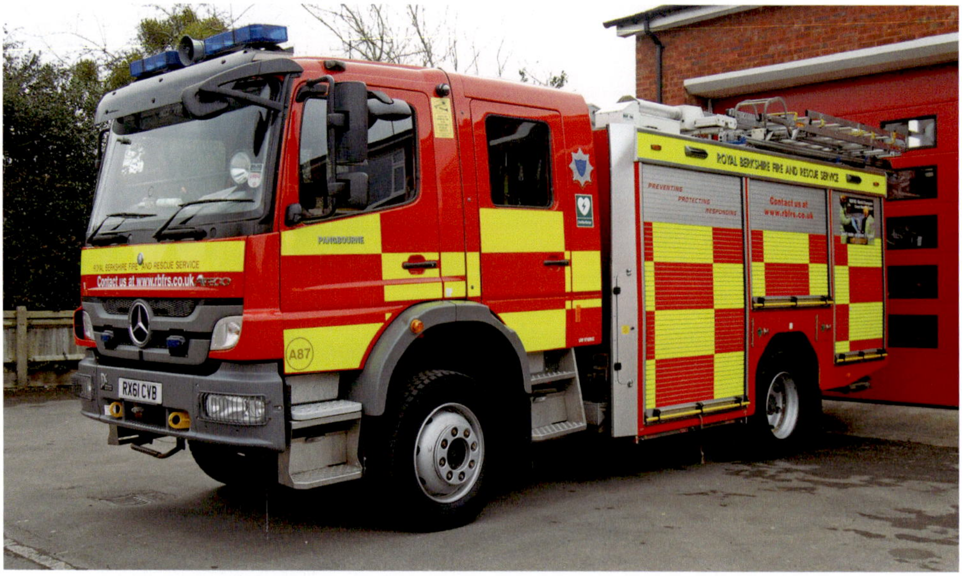

RX61 CVB (2011), one of four Mercedes Atego 4x4/JDC Pump Ladders in the fleet, was the last appliance to serve at Pangbourne. The on-call station was replaced by a new whole-time station in nearby Theale (which also replaced Dee Road Fire Station in the west of Reading); both sites have been demolished and redeveloped for housing. At the time of writing, the 4x4 PLs are stationed at Crowthorne, Hungerford, Maidenhead and Mortimer.

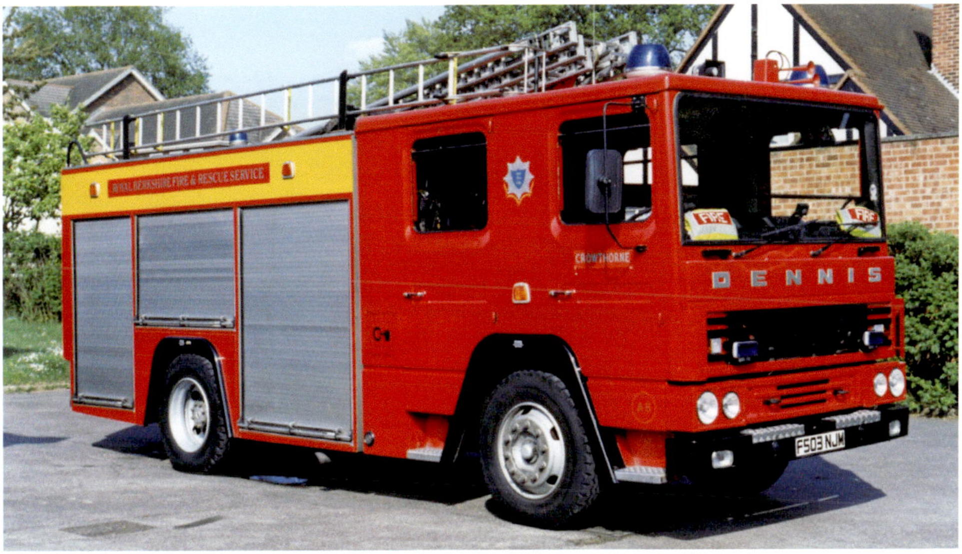

From the early eighties to the mid-nineties, the mainstay of the pumping appliance fleet in Royal Berkshire was the Dennis RS. The first were bodied by Dennis, followed by Locomotors, Carmichael and Reynolds Boughton. An example from the 1988 batch is this Pump Ladder at Crowthorne. F503 NJM had bodywork built by Locomotors on a Dennis RS237 chassis. Just over thirty Dennis RS appliances were purchased by RBF&RS before the chassis was superseded by the Dennis Sabre.

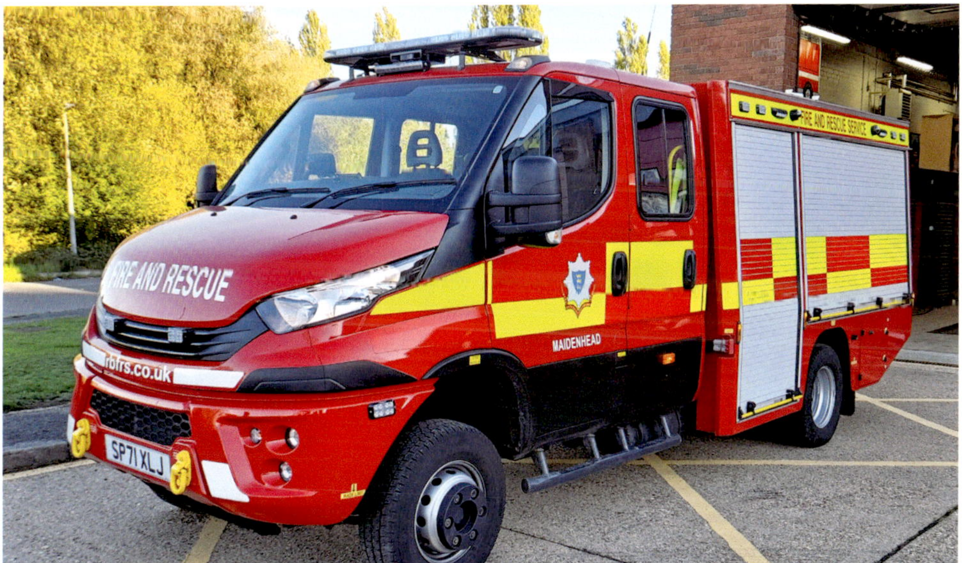

Call-sign One Nine Mike One is a Light 4x4 Pump (L4P) based at Maidenhead Fire Station. SP71 XLJ (2021) is an Iveco Daily 4x4 chassis bodied by Emergency One. Powered by a 3.0-litre diesel engine, the L4P is fitted with a Godiva KP2A multi-pressure pump, a 1,000-litre water tank, high-pressure hose-reel and a range of firefighting and rescue equipment, and can carry a crew of four.

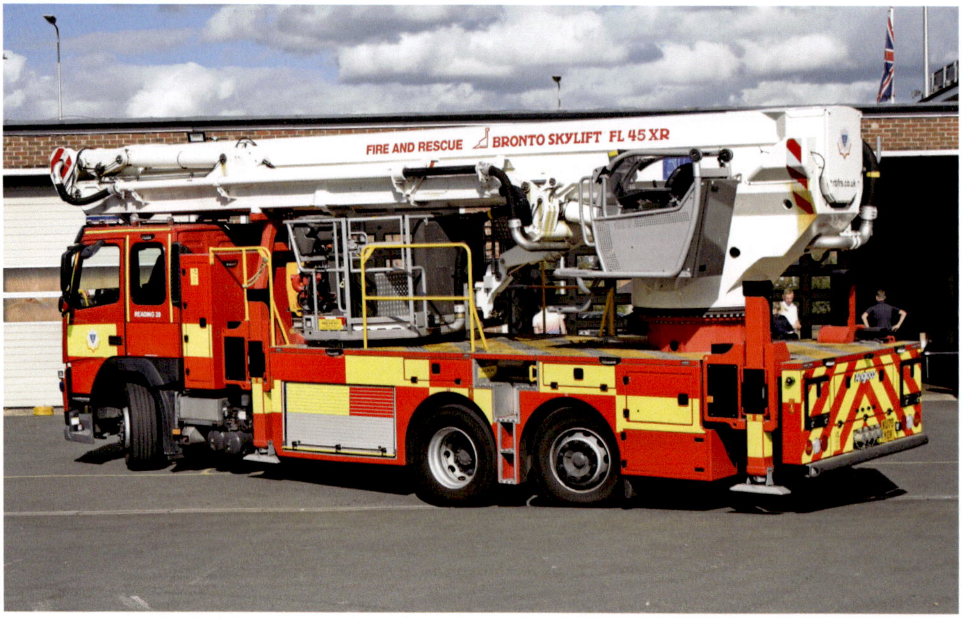

Manoeuvring in the yard of Newbury Fire Station was Royal Berkshire's aerial ladder platform (ALP), which is based at Whitley Wood Fire Station in the south of Reading. KU70 YOV (2020), call-sign Two Zero Alpha One, is a Volvo FM/Angloco/Bronto FL45XR; the 45-metre (135-foot) extended reach booms were mounted on a three-axle chassis with rear wheel steering. This aerial appliance replaced an ALP built on a Mercedes Econic three-axle chassis.

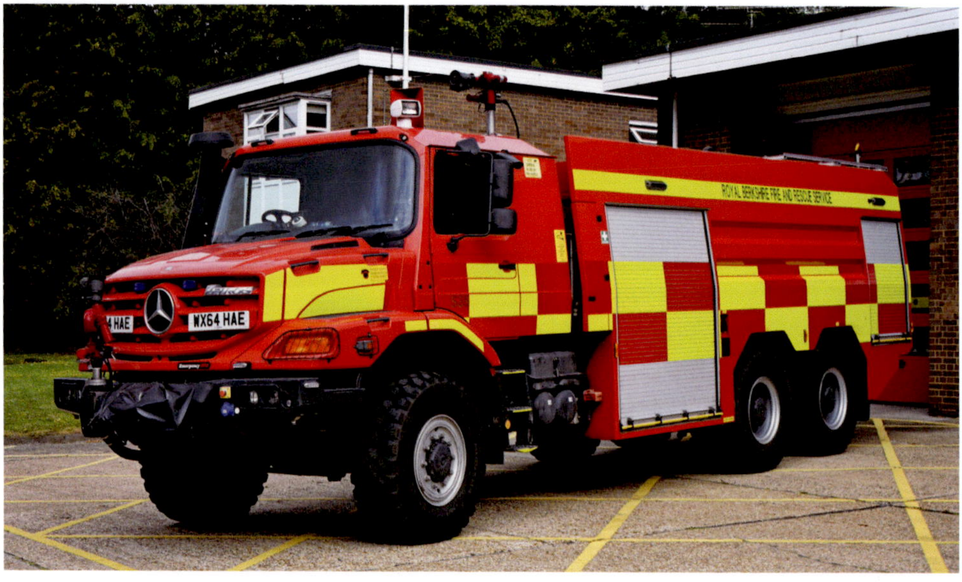

One of the largest water carriers in the UK is Bracknell's Mercedes Zetros 6x6/Emergency One, all-terrain appliance, bought following lessons learnt after the protracted Swinley Forest fire in May 2011. WX64 HAE (2014), fleet number S35, call-sign One Six Whiskey One, carries 8,000 litres of water and 1,000 litres of foam, is fitted with two monitors, spray nozzles and can pump water while moving (similar to airport fire appliances).

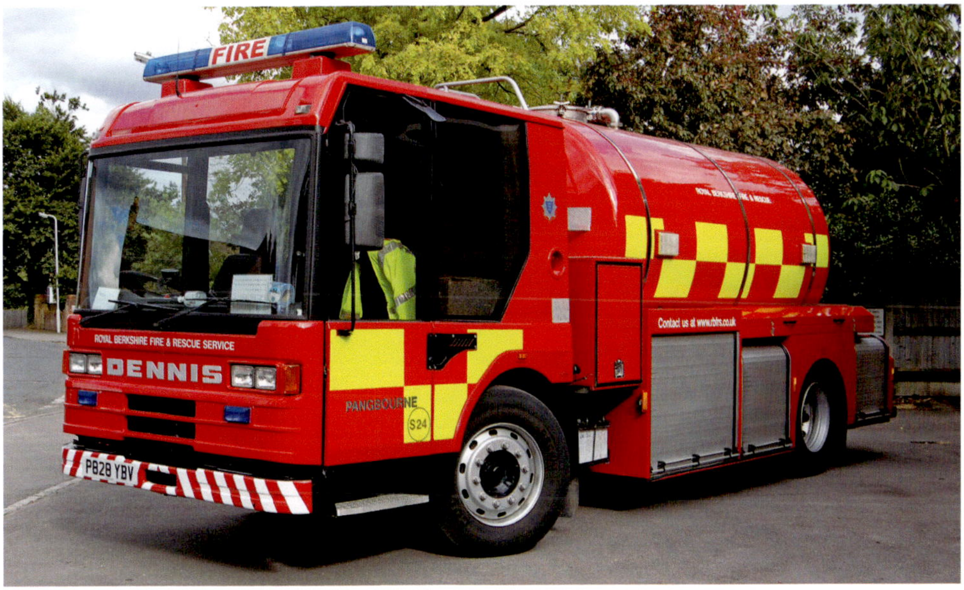

Originally built as a refuse vehicle, P828 YBV (1997), a Dennis Elite chassis, was rebuilt as a water carrier in the early 2000s and fitted with a tank by Crossland. Fleet number S24 spent most of its service at Pangbourne. Following the closure of Pangbourne Fire Station, it was transferred to Wokingham Fire Station (where it was garaged in the old fire station, behind the new building), from where it was crewed when required by personnel from Crowthorne Fire Station.

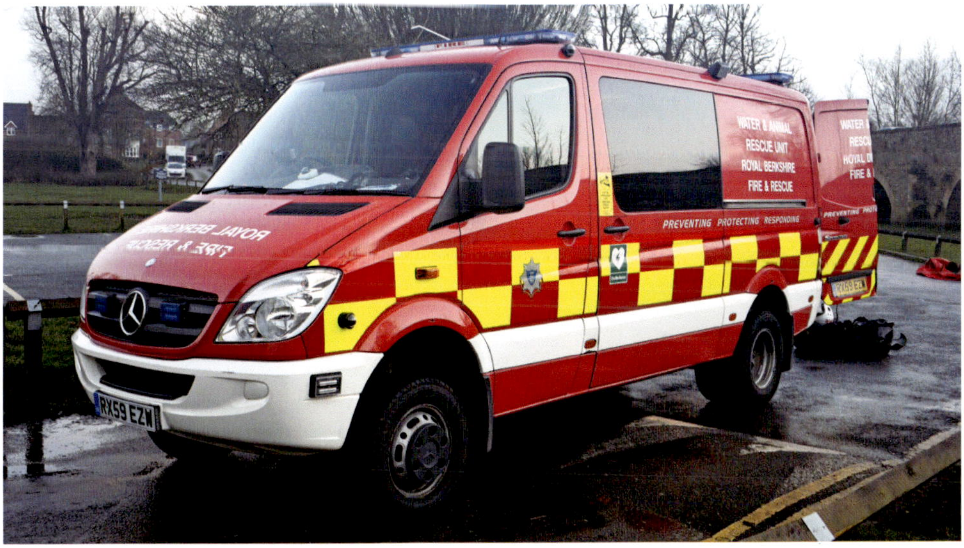

RX59 EZW (2009) is a Mercedes Sprinter 4x4 combi van used as a Water and Animal Rescue Unit (call-sign Zero One Romeo One), which usually tows a rigid boat on a trailer (call-sign Zero One Bravo One), based at Caversham Road Fire Station in Reading (which celebrated its eighty-fifth anniversary in 2024). It was photographed on the Crowmarsh side of the River Thames in Oxfordshire, attending to a narrowboat which had collided with the north side of Wallingford Bridge on 27 December 2022.

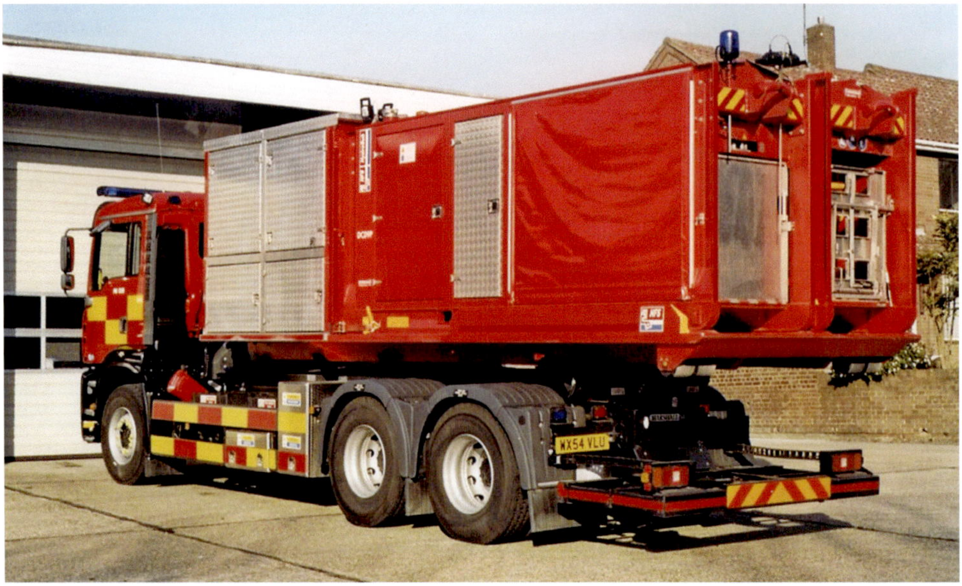

As part of the New Dimensions programme, one of the first High Volume Pumping Units to enter service in the UK was based at Bracknell. Two modules are mounted on a pod, carried on a M.A.N. TGA 26.363 6x4/Marshall prime mover. The modules contain a HydroSub pump, diesel-hydraulic power unit, submersible pump, hose recovery units, 3 km (1.9 miles) of 150-mm (6-inch) hose and ancillary equipment. In the Thames Valley, Bracknell and Banbury each have a pair of PM and HVPU/hose pods.

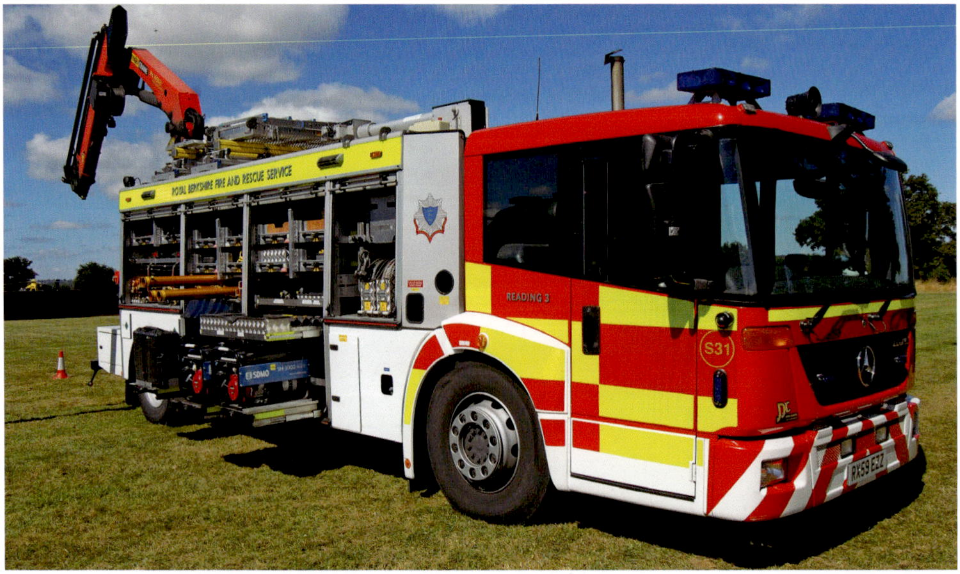

Initially allocated to Newbury, then Dee Road and now at Theale is Royal Berkshire's Heavy Rescue Unit, call-sign Two Two Romeo One. RX59 EZZ (2009), fleet number S31, was built by JDC on a Mercedes Econic chassis with variable height suspension. A Palfinger PK16502 crane is mounted at the rear. Stowed on the roof, behind the telescopic light-mast, is a folding rescue/work platform.

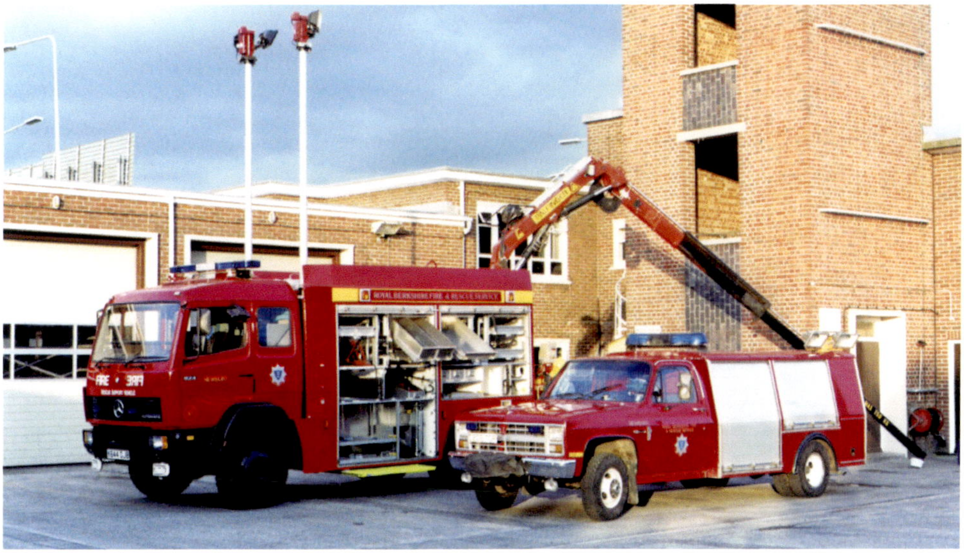

The (then) new and old Rescue Support Vehicles at Newbury were seen together one sunny Friday evening in July 1993. Undergoing crew training was the new RSV, K644 DJB (1992), a Mercedes 1124 4x4, bodied by Locomotors and fitted with two light-masts and a Palfinger crane at the rear. The operational RSV, C206 TDP (1986), a Chevrolet K30 4x4, also bodied by Locomotors, was initially based at Dee Road Fire Station. When on the run, either appliance used the call-sign Alpha Four Five.

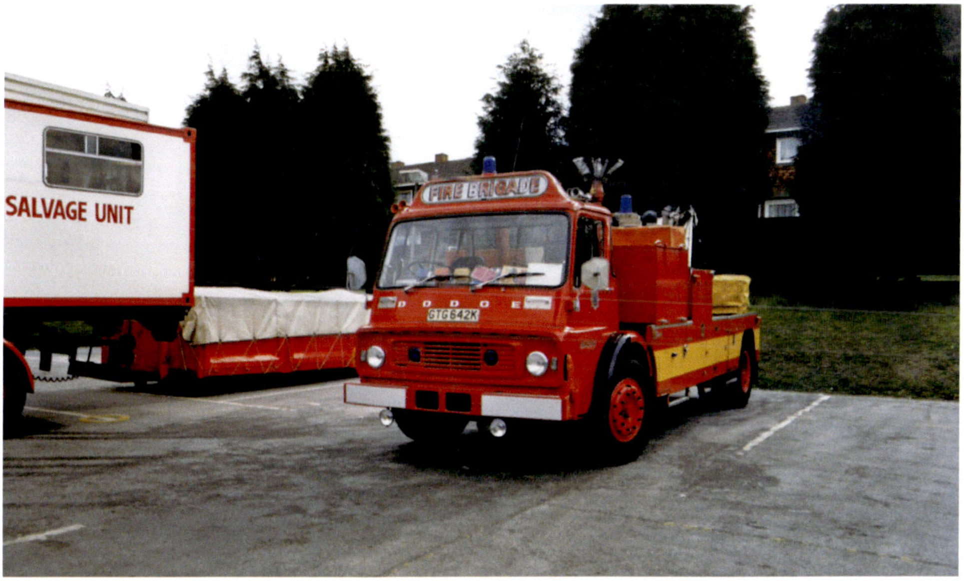

Photographed moments before turning-out from Dee Road to a Road Traffic Accident (as they were known then) on the M4 motorway, on a Saturday afternoon in April 1986, was the ex-Berkshire and Reading Fire Brigade Heavy Rescue Vehicle. GTG 642K (1972), a Dodge K1050, was built by Bates and fitted with Holmes heavy lifting/towing booms. The HRV had a Glamorgan (South Wales) registration (the TG letters), rather than a Reading one. The County of Avon Fire Brigade had a similar HRV.

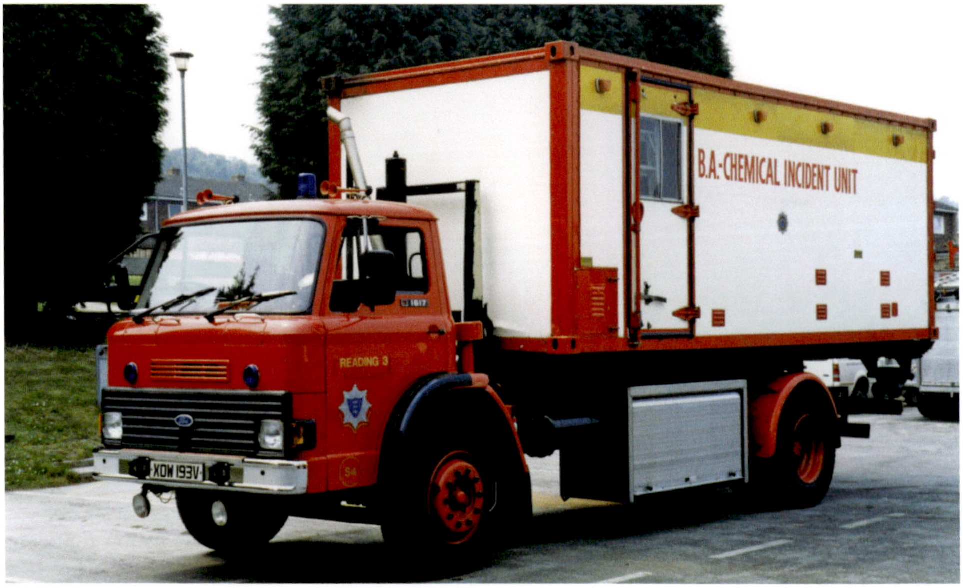

In the late 1970s, the Royal Berkshire Fire Brigade bought several pumping appliances, two turntable ladders and three prime movers based on Ford D series chassis (built locally in Langley). Based at Dee Road during the 1980s was this Ford D1617/Acoma prime mover, carrying a Breathing Apparatus/Chemical Incident Unit pod built by Wilsdon; a number of pods replaced two Special Unit appliances from the 1960s. Thames Valley Police also had two similar but white-liveried Ford D/Powell Duffryn PM to carry a communications pod.

EMFS

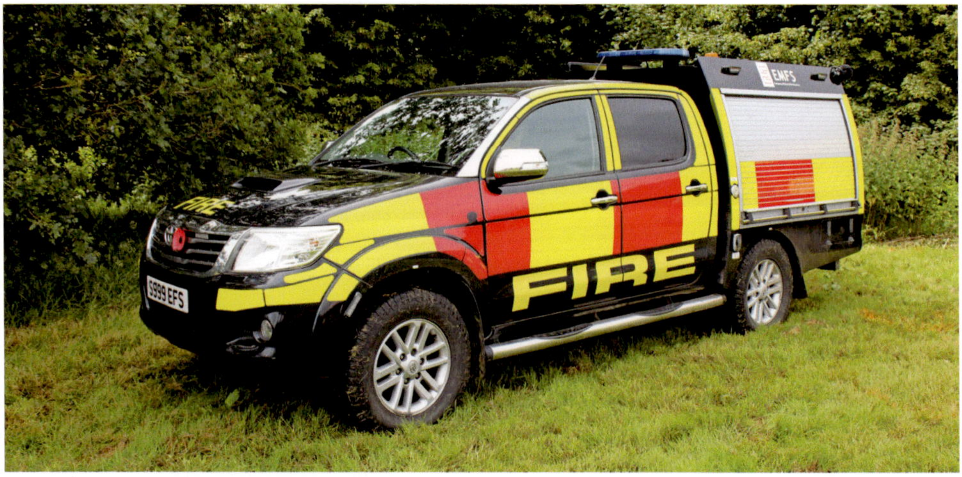

Based in Oxfordshire, EMFS (Emergency, Medical and Fire Solutions) operates a fleet of ambulances and fire appliances providing cover for events across the UK. Providing fire cover at the Thames Valley Air Ambulance's 25th Anniversary Big Birthday Bash event held at the Penn House Estate in Buckinghamshire in June 2024 was this appliance in a black livery. S999 EFS (2014) is a Toyota HiLux 4x4 double cab with bodywork by Pick-Up Systems. (Photo: Gethin Roberts)

HOME OFFICE

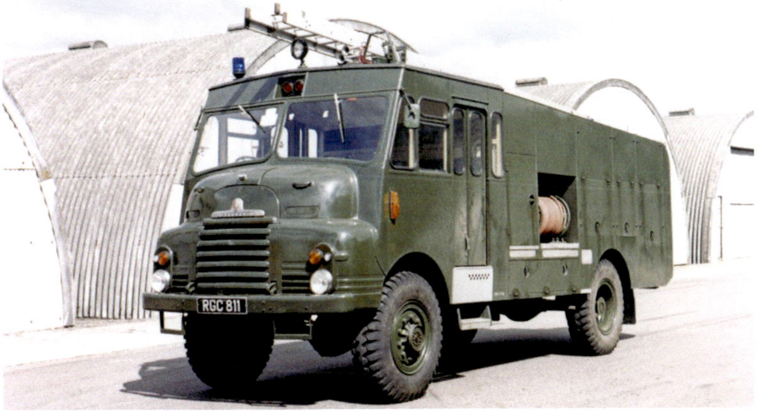

Originally built as self-propelled pumps for use by the Auxiliary Fire Service (which was disbanded in 1968) to pump large quantities of water following a nuclear attack, over 3,000 Emergency Pumps (or 'Green Goddesses', as they were nicknamed) were built and later stored at locations across the UK. Around 900 were then stored at a depot in Staffordshire before disposal in the mid-2000s. Seen at the former Home Office stores at Steventon in Oxfordshire in 1990 was RGC 811 (1956), a Bedford RLHZ 4x4. The bodywork of the EPs was built by various firms.

ROYAL AIR FORCE/DEFENCE FIRE & RESCUE SERVICE

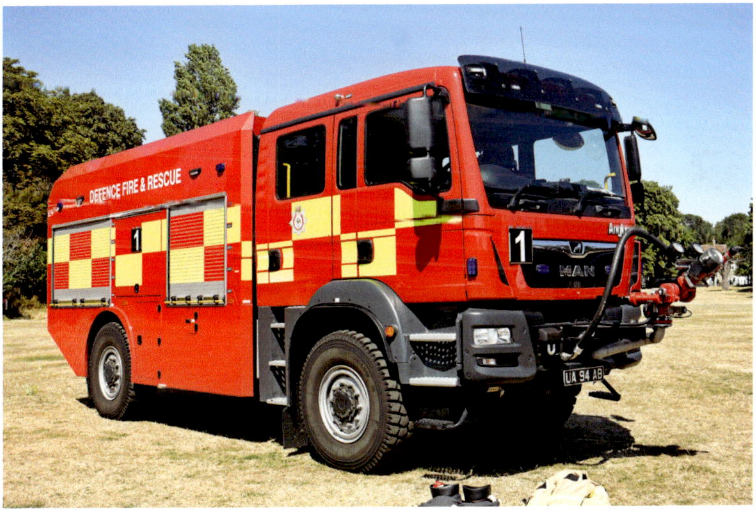

RAF Benson in the south of Oxfordshire is home to helicopters of the Joint Helicopter Command and also hosts a National Police Air Service helicopter and the Thames Valley Air Ambulance helicopter. Among the appliances providing fire and rescue cover is UA 94 AB (2021), a MAN 4x4/Angloco Multi-Purpose Response Vehicle, which can be used for aviation or structural firefighting and rescue. It was photographed on display on The Kinecroft recreation field in Wallingford in July 2022.

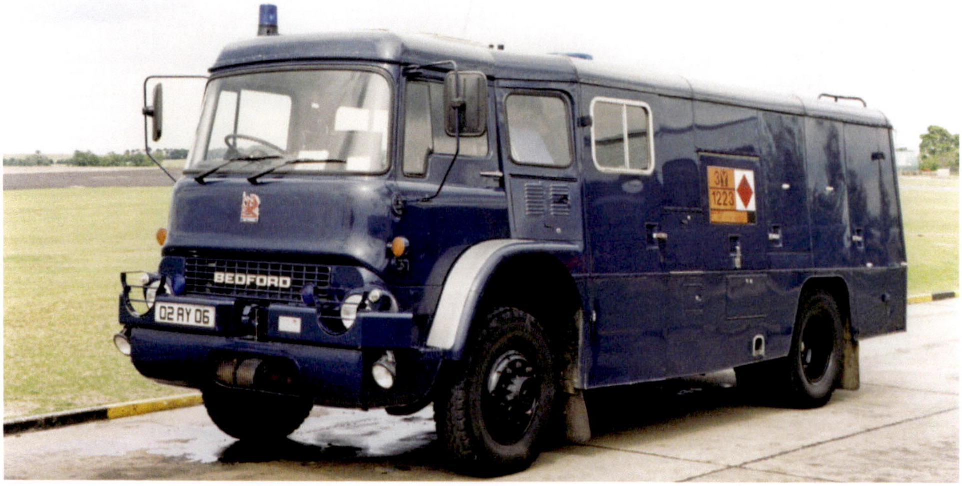

The Queen's Flight of the Royal Air Force was based at RAF Benson, until reforming at RAF Northolt as No. 32 (The Royal) Squadron in 1995. To support helicopter flights at non-airfield locations, the Queen's Flight operated three Range Rover 6x4 TACR2 and three Bedford M1120 4x4/Edgehill, Helicopter Support Vehicles (HSV), all painted blue. In addition to carrying firefighting and rescue equipment, the HSVs carried aviation fuel (as indicated by the Hazchem warning signs). 02 AY 06 was seen at Benson in 1990. The HSVs were replaced by Scania 4x4 appliances, also painted blue.

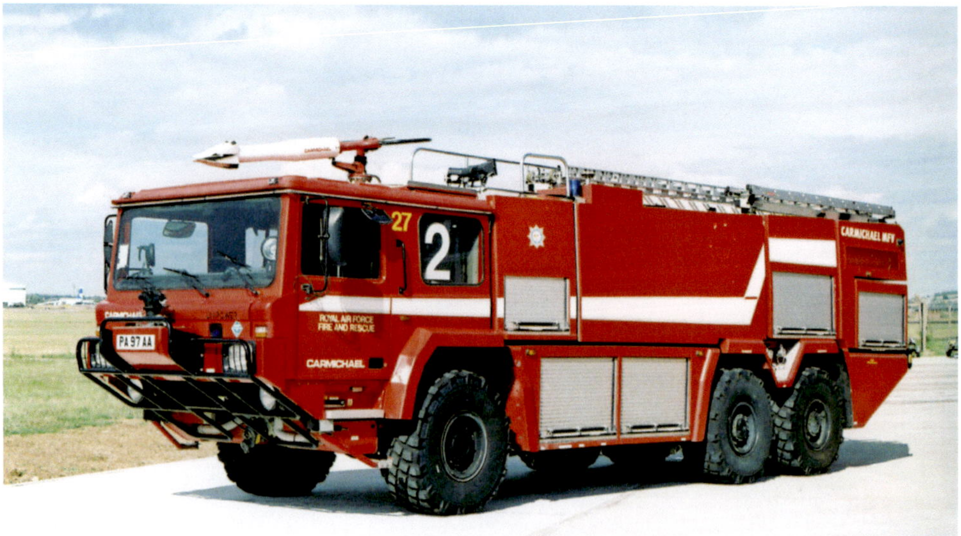

RAF Brize Norton in the west of Oxfordshire is the Royal Air Force's largest station and home to the Air Mobility Force, along with sixteen squadrons and units and its largest aircraft (Airbus A400 Atlas, Airbus A330 Voyager and Boeing C-17 Globemaster). In 2006, one of four Unipower 6x6/Carmichael MFVs (Major Foam Vehicles) was PA 97 AA, built in the late 1990s. MFVs carried 6,819 litres (1,500 gallons) of water, 818 litres (180 gallons) of foam and two x 50 kg (220 lbs) dry powder. The MFVs were replaced by Oshkosh Striker 6x6 appliances.

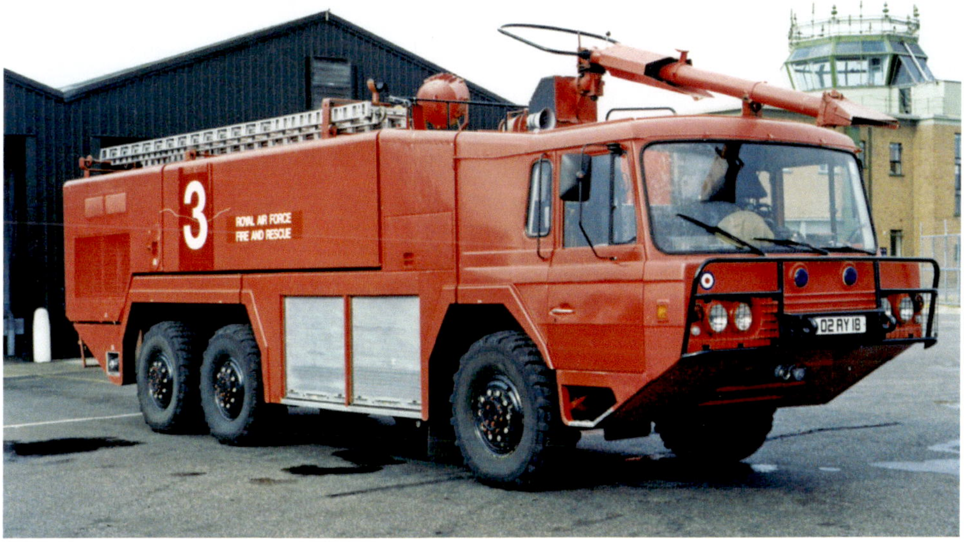

In 1986, the old fire station at RAF Brize Norton had a fleet of five fire appliances in a mix of red and green liveries. Number Three was this Mk.11 crash tender, 02 AY 18 (1985). Built by Gloster Saro on a Scammell Nubian Major 6x6 chassis, it carried 5,683 litres (1,250 gallons) of water, 682 litres (150 gallons) of foam and 100 kg (220 lbs) BCF. There was also one Mk.11A, fitted with a hydraulic ladder and cage for reaching the tail-mounted engine of the Tri-Star aircraft in service with the RAF at the time.

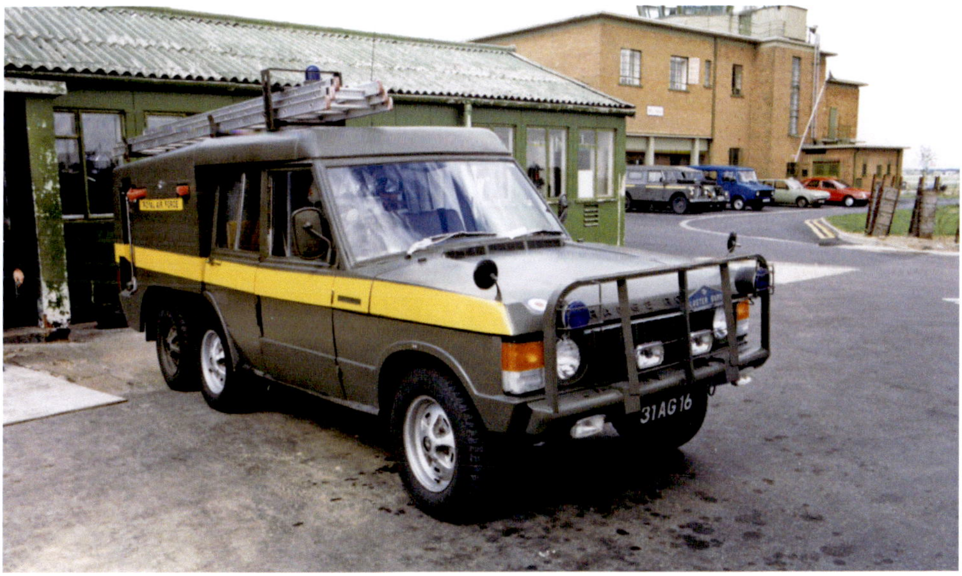

Also at Brize Norton was 31 AG 16, one of a large number of TACR2 (Truck, Airfield Crash Rescue, Mk.2) built by Gloster Saro in the late 1970s. Based on the Range Rover 4x4 chassis (which then only had two doors), a third non-powered axle, rear crew cab doors, bodywork, light-mast, pump and tank were fitted. A small number were built by HCB-Angus in the late 1980s, while Carmichael built the Mk.2A version.

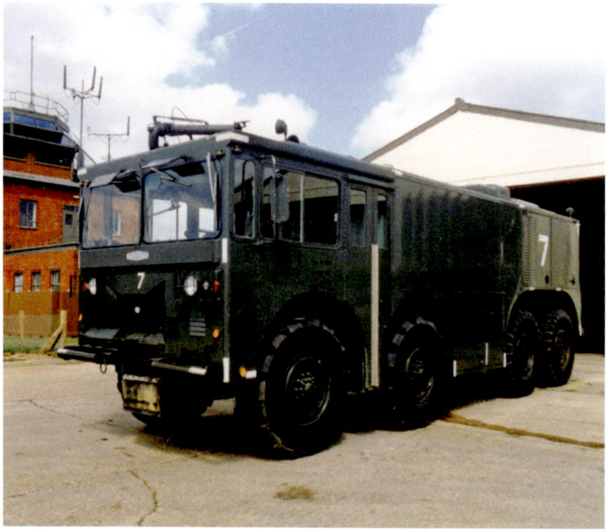

Unit 7 at RAF Greenham Common in Berkshire in 1988 was built by FWD as a P2 type crash truck. The 8x8 chassis had two water/foam monitors, carried 2,300 US gallons (8,706 litres) of water, 200 US gallons (757 litres) of foam and had a 1,400 US gallons per minute (5,300 litres per minute) pump. Overhauled by Quality in the early 1980s, they were re-designated P2A. Although the airfield fire station has been demolished, the neighbouring control tower is now a visitor centre (one display includes information on the USAF FD) and the former domestic/technical site fire station is now used by a small business.

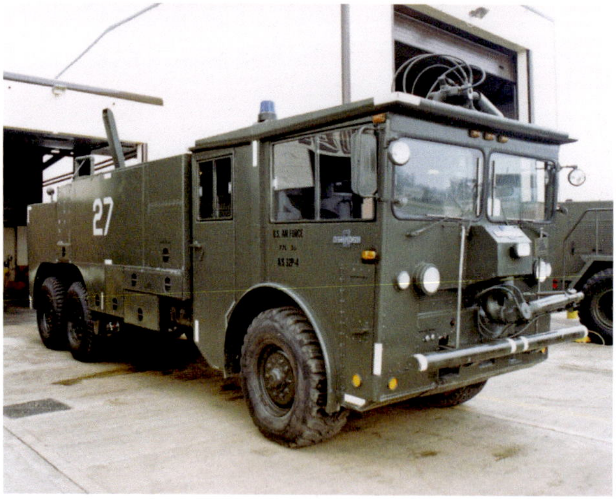

In 1991, Unit 27 at RAF Upper Heyford in Oxfordshire was a 1977 Oshkosh 6x6/Oshkosh, P4 type crash truck (77 L 26) fitted with both roof-mounted and front-mounted water/foam monitors, carrying 1,500 US gallons (5,678 litres) of water, 200 US gallons (757 litres) of foam and had a 1,000 US gallons per minute (3,785 litres per minute) pump. Upper Heyford played a brief role in the 1983 James Bond film *Octopussy* as the fictitious Feldstadt Air Force Base in West Germany.

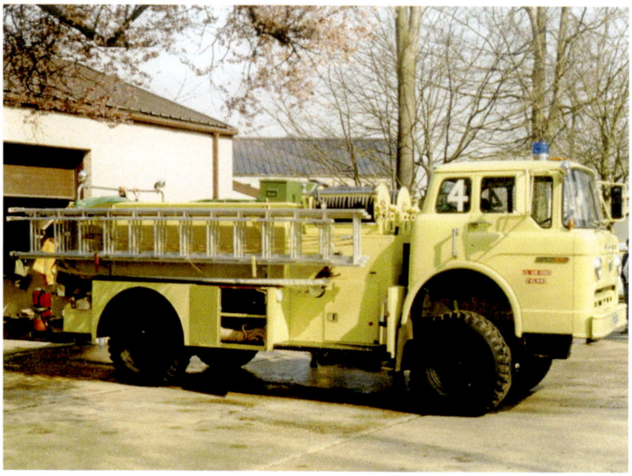

Compared to the USAF's airfields in the UK, one American base that was relatively unknown was RAF Daws Hill in Buckinghamshire, located in the suburbs of High Wycombe, close to the M40 motorway. This small, non-flying base was in use between the early 1940s and mid-1990s. When visited in the early 1990s, there were only around 350 US military and civilian personnel on the base, including a small fire crew operating a 1974 Ford C 4x4/Ward La France, P8 type pumper (74 L 943) and a Freight Rover Sherpa 250 GPV. (Photo: the late Ray Roberts)

Chapter 3
Miscellaneous Emergency Services

In addition to the three main emergency services, several other organisations operate vehicles which respond to incidents within the Thames Valley and beyond.

Some of the organisations and vehicles featured are unique to the Thames Valley, while similar organisations and vehicles can be found in other parts of the United Kingdom.

While some of the organisations have full-time staff and are publicly funded, many rely on volunteers and donations.

The work of these organisations is diverse and varies from supporting the three main emergency services, providing emergency medical support, healthcare, explosive ordnance disposal, supporting the survivors of serious incidents; emergency planning, preparedness, resilience and response; protecting the environment; lowland search and rescue; responding to incidents on roads and railways or involving aircraft; providing security and supporting sporting events.

Some of the organisations featured no longer operate in the Thames Valley and some of the vehicles featured have long since been disposed of but as with older vehicles in the other chapters, they are included for historical interest.

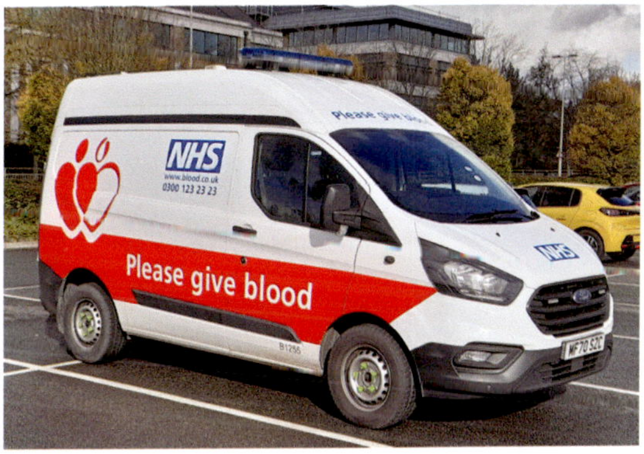

NHS Blood & Transplant provides a blood and transplantation service to the NHS, running blood donation services in England and transplant services across the UK. The NHS B&T Logistics Department has a fleet of 220 vehicles, some fitted with blue lights and sirens for urgent deliveries. This Ford Transit Custom van, MF70 SZC (2020), was seen in Bracknell in 2022.

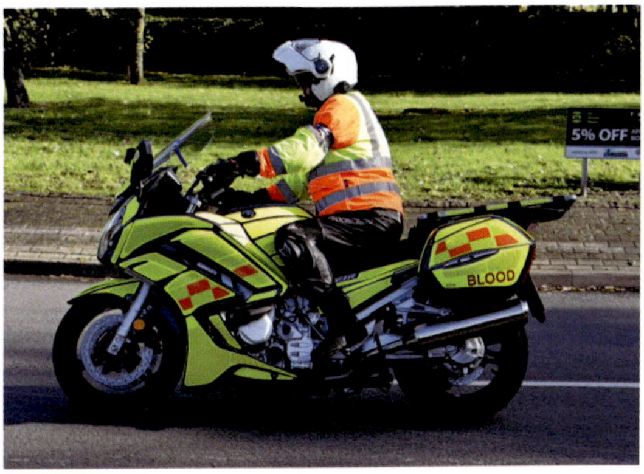

Also taking part in the Ride of Respect 2019 was this Yamaha FJR 1300 of SERV OBN (Service by Emergency Rider Volunteers – Oxon, Bucks, Berks and Northants). The charity provides an out-of-hours rapid response transport service free of charge to the NHS, carrying blood and blood products plus other urgently required items. The team has a fleet of Yamaha FJR 1300 and BMW F800 GT motorcycles, all named after women who have made a significant contribution to medicine.

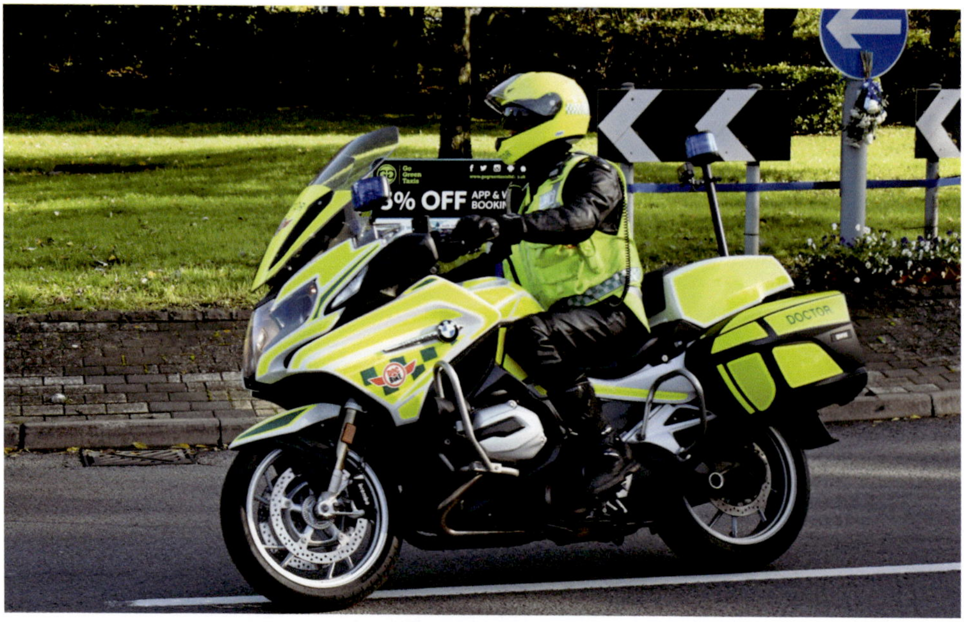

Another emergency medical motorcycle taking part in the Ride of Respect 2019 was this BMW R1200 RT from the Doc Bike charity. Doc Bike was founded in Dorset in 2013 and has teams in Avon & Somerset, Cheshire, Devon, Dorset, Northamptonshire, North Wales, Staffordshire and Sussex. Working with air ambulance charities and the emergency services, Doc Bike provides roadside critical care, injury prevention and supports the Biker Down and Bike Safe schemes.

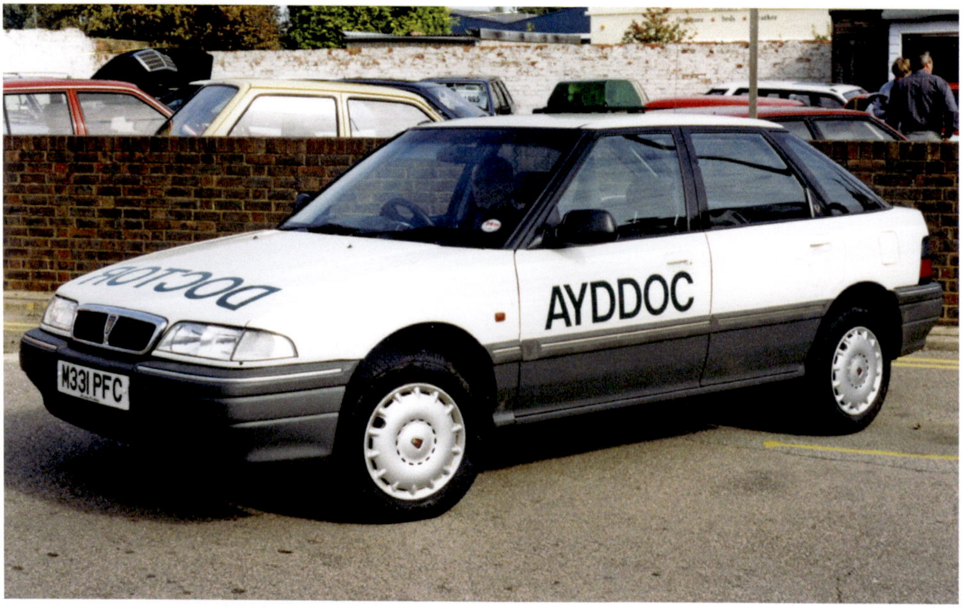

AYDDOC (Aylesbury District Doctors), an out-of-hours general practitioner co-operative, was formed in Buckinghamshire in 1994. Seen at the former Aylesbury Fire Station in Cambridge Street in 1996 were two Rover 218D hatchbacks. M331 PFC was new in 1994 and both cars (M332 PFC was the other) were being driven by off-duty firefighters.

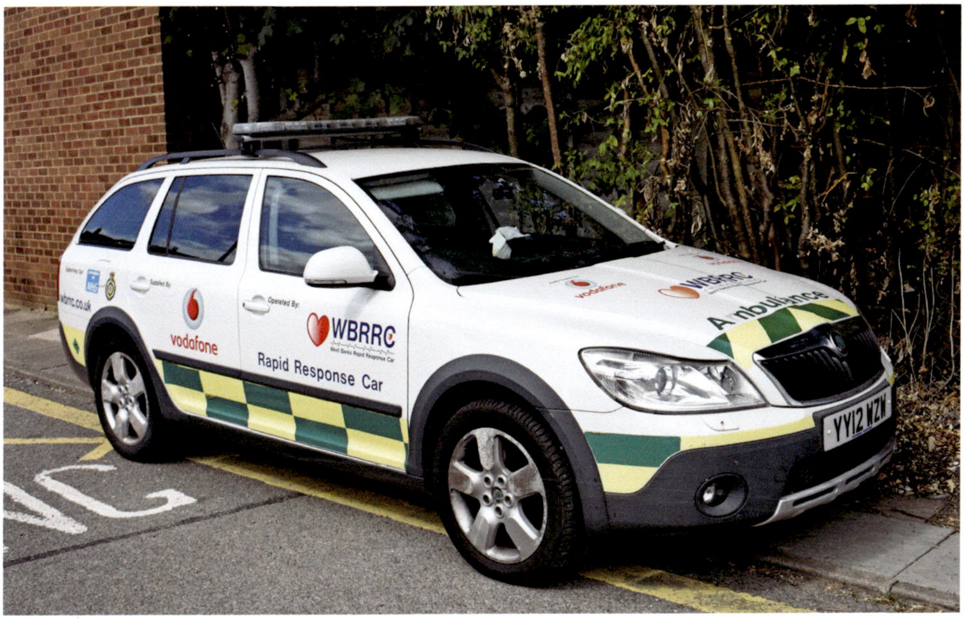

Seen at Newbury Fire Station's open day in 2022 was YY12 WZW (2012), a Skoda Octavia Scout 4x4 Rapid Response Car. This is one of a small fleet of four Skoda cars used by off-duty paramedics and technicians to attend serious medical emergencies in West Berkshire. The West Berkshire Rapid Response Cars charity was set up in 2004 and has previously used Volkswagen cars.

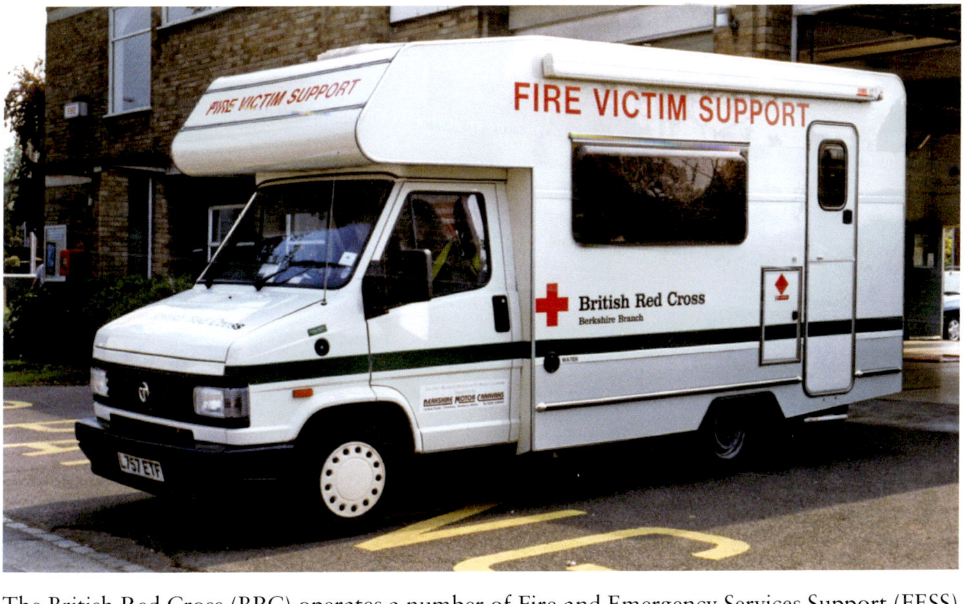

The British Red Cross (BRC) operates a number of Fire and Emergency Services Support (FESS) teams across the UK. One of the first teams to be formed was in the Berkshire Branch of the BRC in 1993. The team of volunteers respond to residential property fires to provide practical and emotional support to fire victims. L757 ETF, a 1993 Talbot Express/Richard Holdsworth motor-home, was based for many years at Wokingham Road Fire Station in the east of Reading.

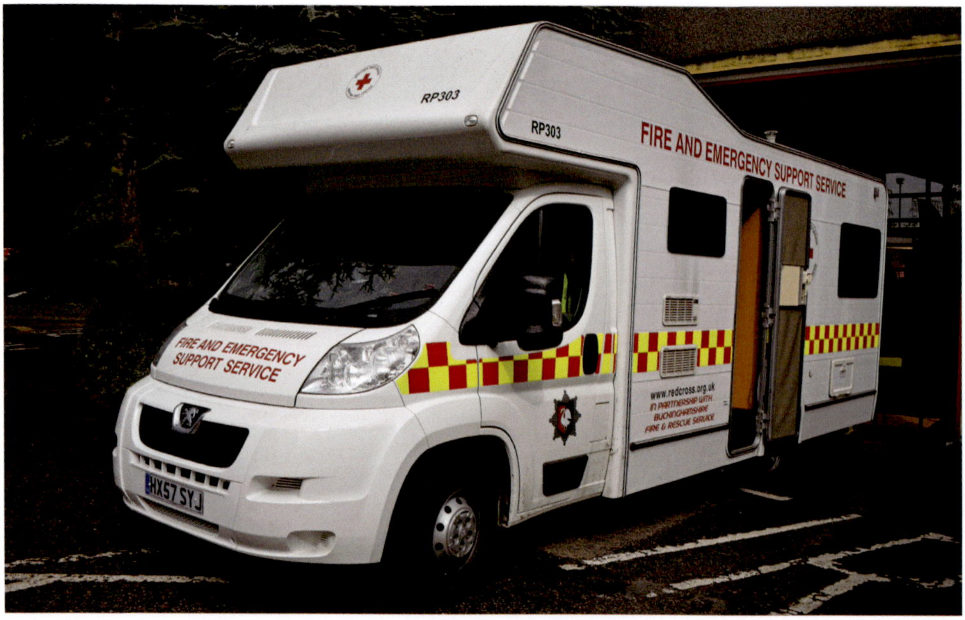

On display at the open day at the former Bletchley Fire Station in 2017 was HX57 SYJ, a 2008 Peugeot Boxer motor home of the Buckinghamshire Branch of the BRC. This vehicle replaced Y881 FTW, a 2001-built motor home also based on a Peugeot Boxer chassis. The Oxfordshire branch of the BRC also has a FESS team based at Rewley Road Fire Station in the centre of Oxford.

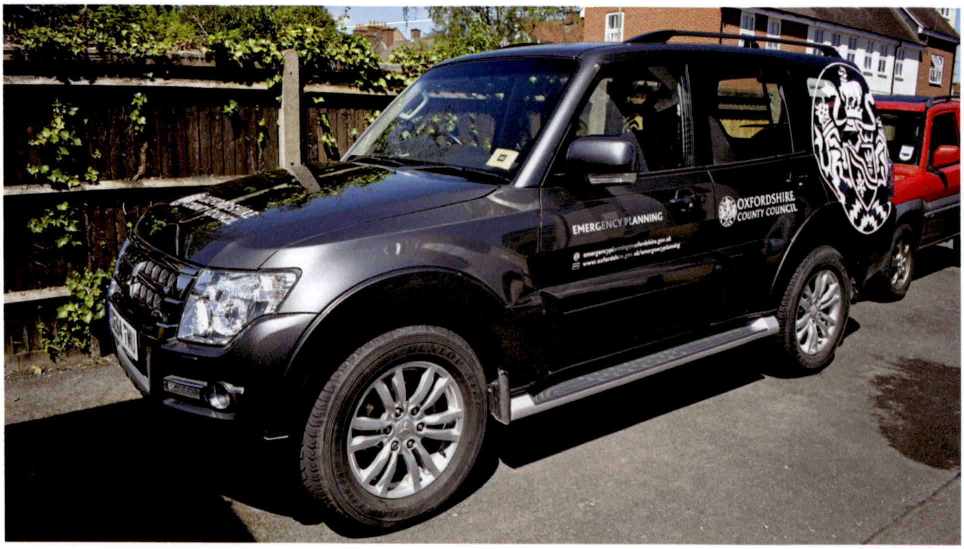

Local authorities have statutory duties under the Civil Contingencies Act 2004 to ensure that they are prepared for and able to respond to incidents. This work includes assessing risks; writing, reviewing and exercising emergency plans; working with emergency services, national organisations and operators of major risk sites; and providing advice to local communities and businesses. Seen at Abingdon Fire Station open day in 2018 was Oxfordshire County Council's Emergency Planning Unit's Mitsubishi Shogun 4x4 vehicle OE64 TMU (2015).

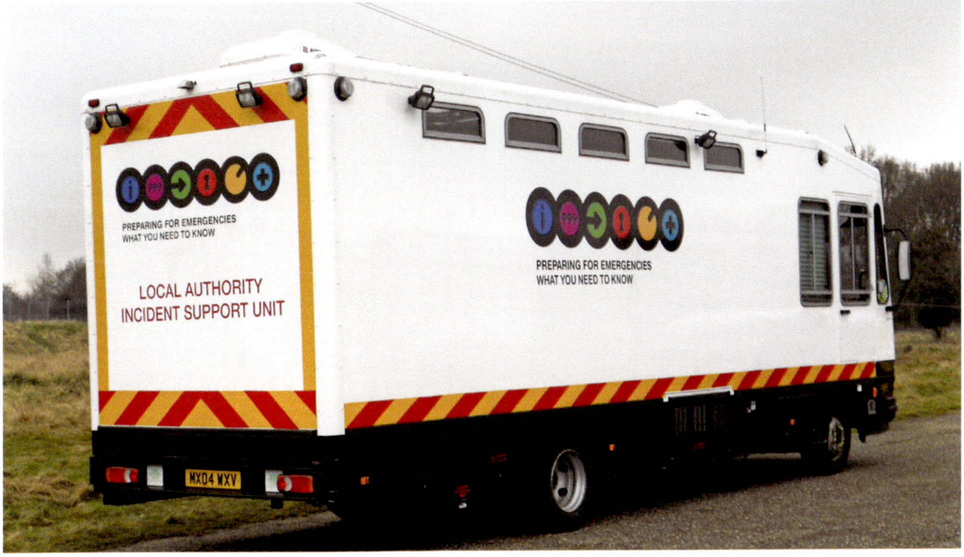

West Berkshire Council's Emergency Planning Unit had this mobile-library-style ISU vehicle, MX04 WXV (2004), built on a Daf LF 45.150 chassis, at an exercise in 2013. Exercise Counterpart took place at the now closed Aborfield Garrison (since redeveloped for housing), to test the concept of a Radiation Monitoring Unit being set up to monitor people following an incident involving the release of radioactive material; also the setting up of MD1 mass decontamination equipment carried on Incident Response Units from the Royal Berkshire and Oxfordshire F&RSs.

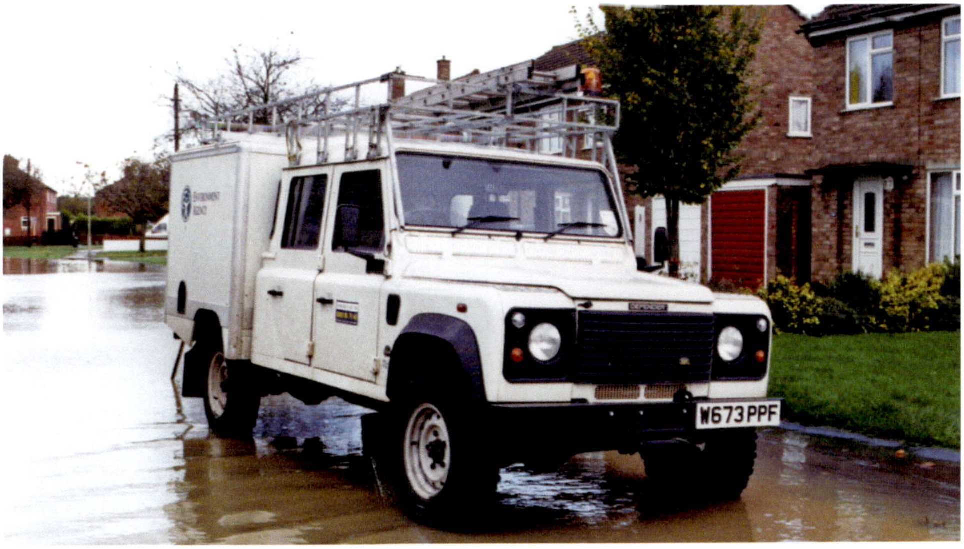

With its headquarters in Bristol, the Environment Agency was formed in 1996 to regulate major industry and waste, the treatment of contaminated land, water quality and resources, fisheries, rivers, conservation and ecology in England. It is also responsible for managing the risk of flooding from rivers. Seen at flooding in the north of Abingdon in 2007 was this 2000 Land Rover 127" crew-cab 4x4, fitted with a front-mounted winch, box body and roof rack. (Photo: the late Ray Roberts)

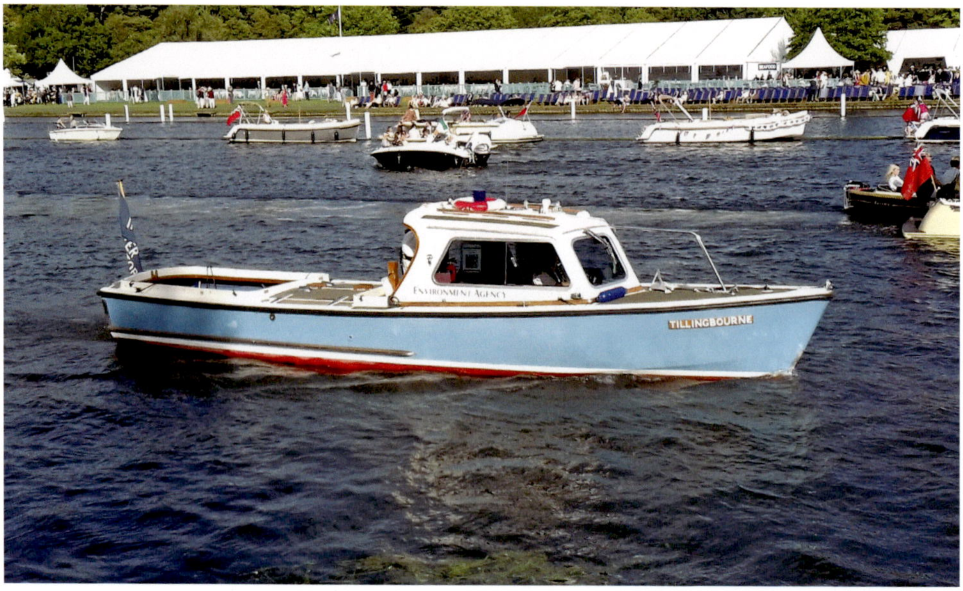

One of five Environment Agency River Inspector's boats patrolling the River Thames between Oxfordshire and Berkshire during the 2021 Henley Royal Regatta was named *Tillingbourne* (a river in Surrey), the other boats being *Chess*, *Ellenbrook*, *Whitewater* and *Wye*. In addition, the Hampshire and Isle of Wight Constabulary's Marine Unit also had a Humber rigid inflatable boat on patrol. The regatta takes place over six days in June and July, with rowing races over a course length of 1 mile, 550 yards (2 km, 112 metres).

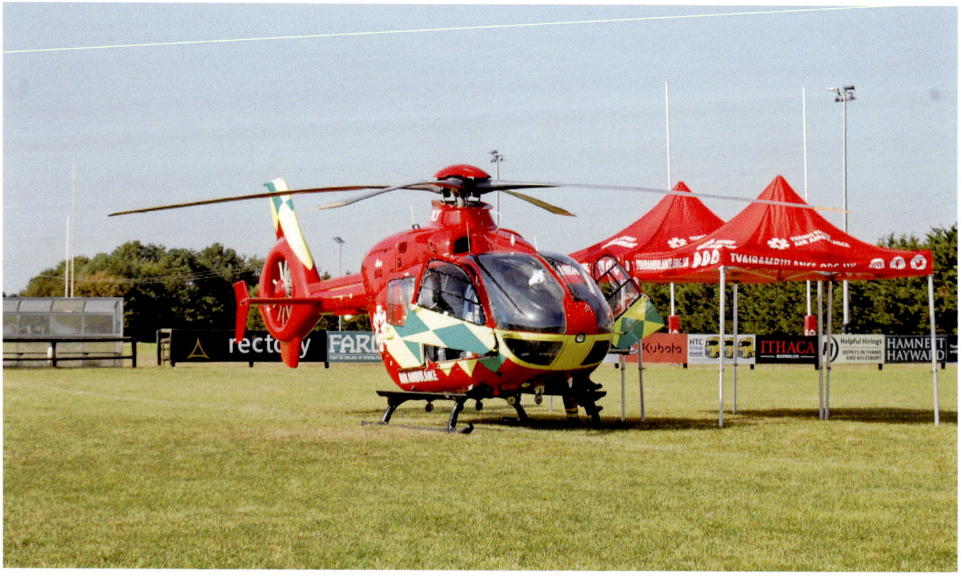

G-TVLY, an Airbus H-135, was previously in service with the Devon Air Ambulance. It is seen here at a fundraising event at Chinnor Rugby Club in Thame, Oxfordshire, on a very hot day in September 2023. The Thames Valley and Chiltern Air Ambulance was established at White Waltham Airfield in Berkshire in 1999, operating an Augusta A109 helicopter. In 2007, the renamed Thames Valley Air Ambulance relocated its flying base to RAF Benson in Oxfordshire.

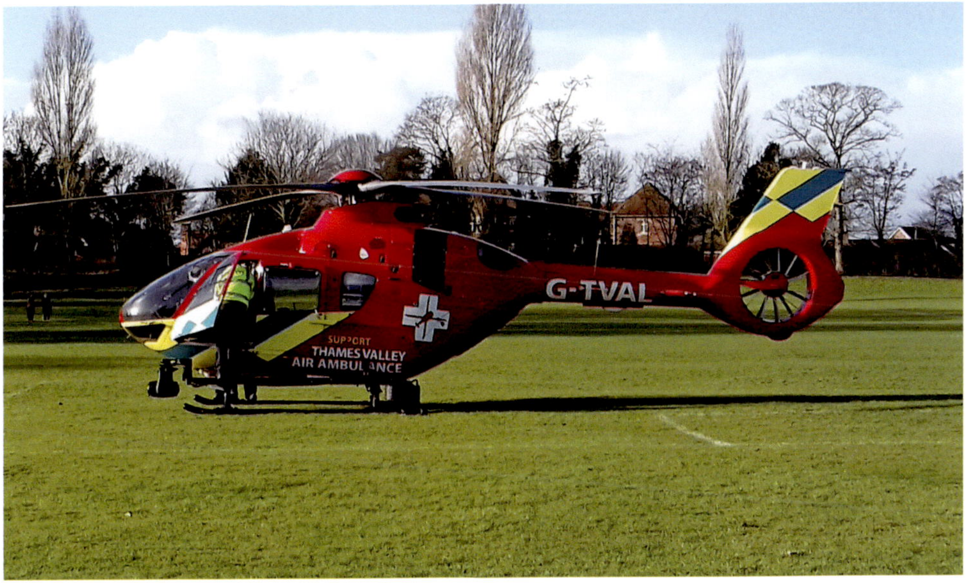

G-TVAL, a Eurocopter EC-135, landed on The Bullcroft recreation field in Wallingford, just a few miles from its base at RAF Benson, during the morning of Saturday 19 December 2020. The pilot had shut down both engines and was waiting for the return of the two medical crew from a call in Wallingford town centre; on this occasion, there was no need to fly a patient to hospital. The helicopter is now in service with the National Ambulance Service in Ireland.

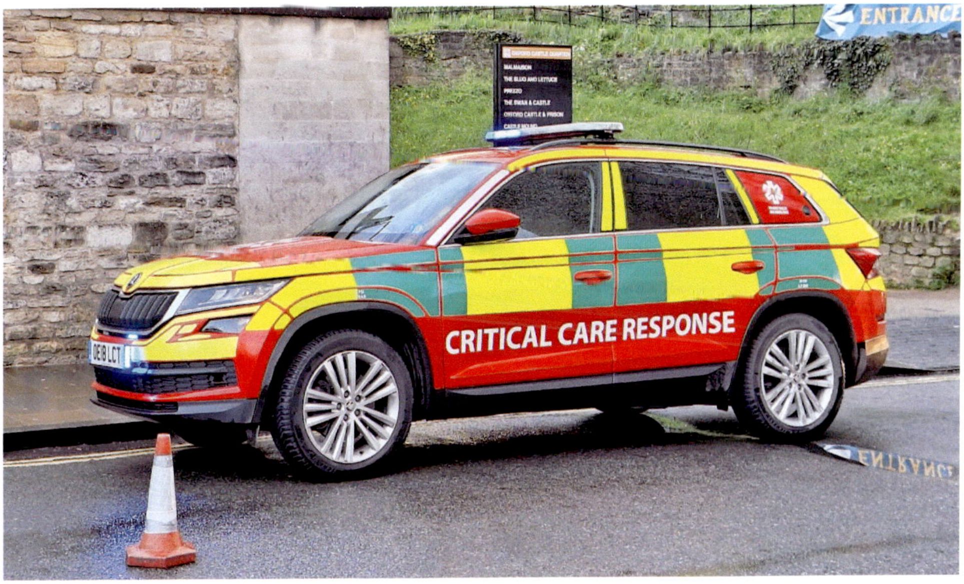

One of five TVAA Critical Care Response Units based on Skoda Kodiaq 4x4 SUVs (which are actually painted blue but are wrapped in their red livery). These vehicles were based with the helicopter at RAF Benson but have moved to the TVAA HQ at Stokenchurch in Buckinghamshire from where they are pre-deployed to locations across the Thames Valley. OE18 LCT (2018) was seen attending a call to the Castle Mound in New Road, Oxford, on 1 April 2024. Also attending were a WrL and HP from the nearby Rewley Road Fire Station. (Photo: Richard Roberts)

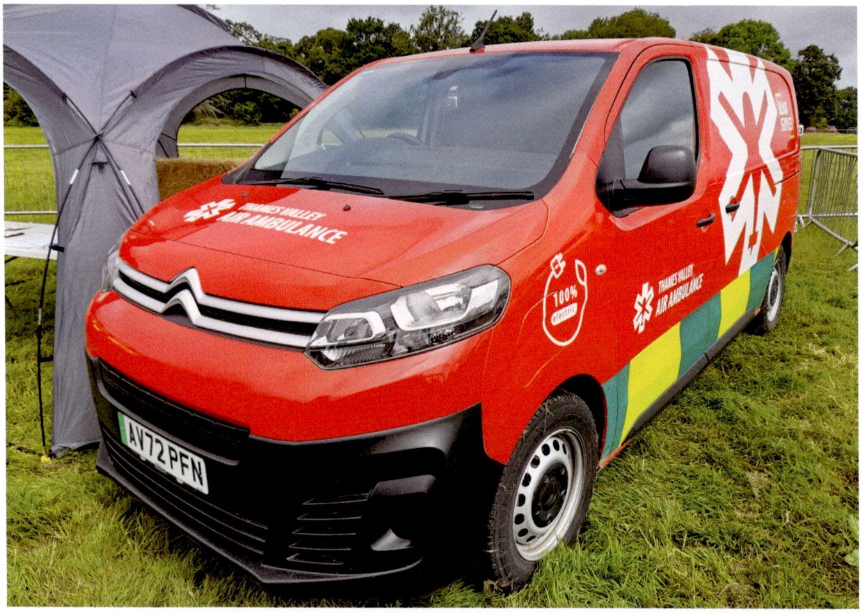

On display at the TVAA 25th Anniversary Event in Penn, Buckinghamshire, in June 2024 was this electric van. AV72 PFN (2022) is a Citroen E-Dispatch which is used daily to replenish the blood supplies carried on the air ambulance and the CCRUs, including red blood cells and fresh frozen plasma. As with the CCRUs, this vehicle has been wrapped in its livery.

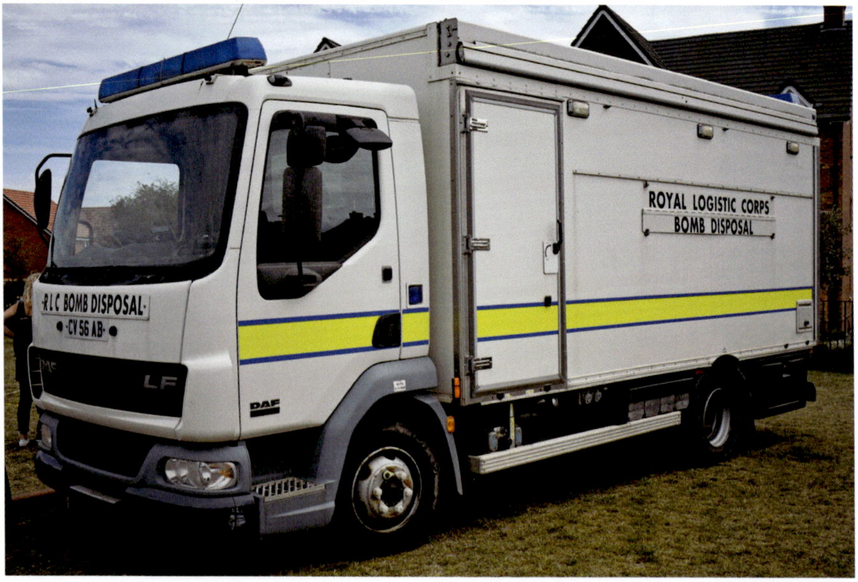

On display at an Emergency Services event in Didcot in 2019 was this Daf LF Explosive Ordnance Disposal (EOD) vehicle. Part of the British Army's Royal Logistics Corps, 11 EOD and Search Regiment has its HQ at Vauxhall Barracks in Didcot. The regiment is divided into five squadrons, which are subdivided into troops based across the UK. Their roles include the disposal of conventional munitions and improvised explosive devices; inspection and licensing of ammunition storage; and enforcing explosives safety regulations.

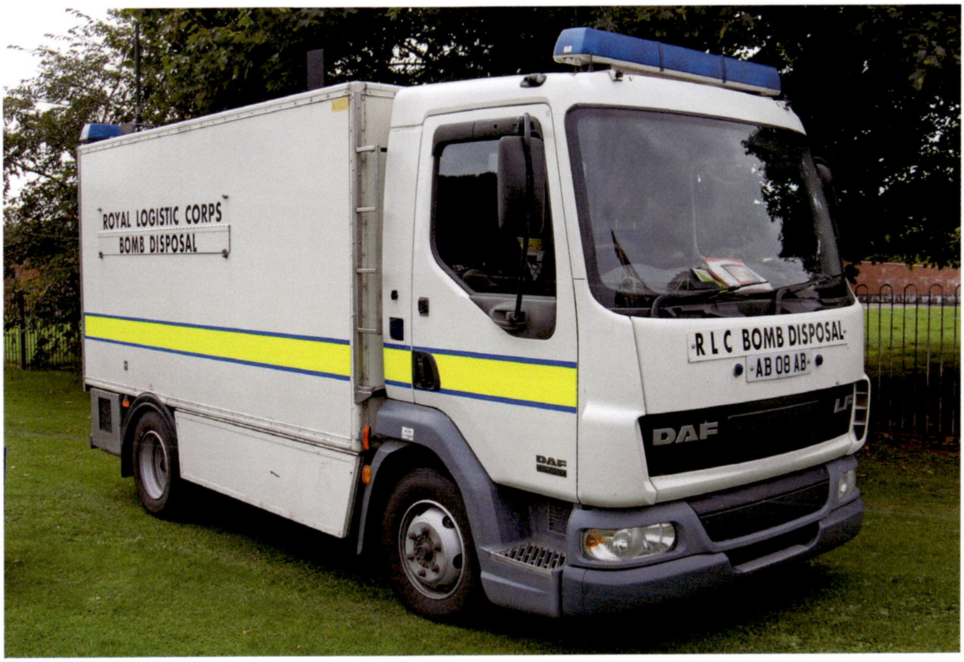

On display at an Emergency Services event in Didcot in 2017 was this Daf LF EOD vehicle of 11 EOD and Search Regiment. Amongst the numerous items of equipment carried is a Cutlass, six-wheeled, remote-controlled robot; the regiment deployed a Cutlass at the scene of the collapse of the boiler house at the former Didcot A Power Station in February 2016. The regiment has a fleet of marked and unmarked vehicles and at the time of writing was undergoing a replacement programme.

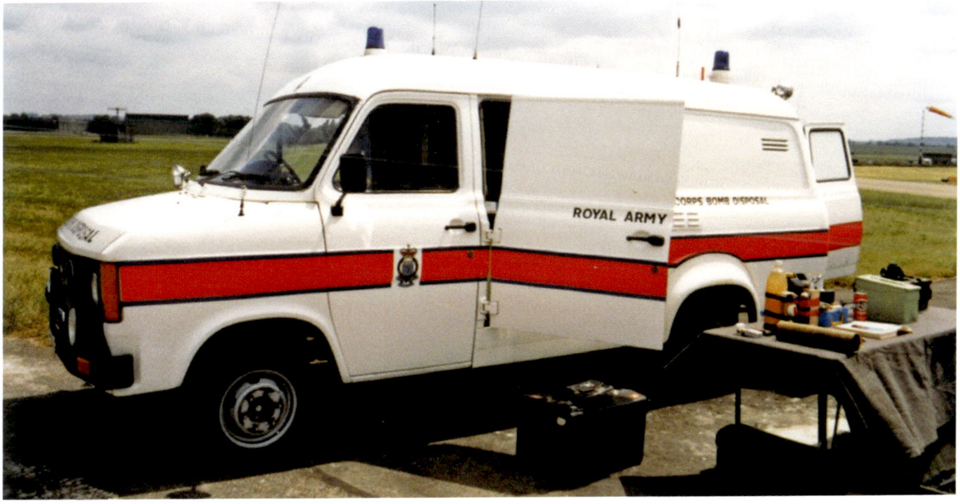

One of the demonstrations at the RAF Benson Families Day in 1988 was by a Royal Army Ordnance Corps, Explosive Ordnance Disposal troop. Behind the display of simulated improvised explosive devices is a Ford Transit Mk.2 LWB van (dating from the late 1970s/early 1980s), carrying a tracked robot, often referred to as a 'wheelbarrow'. In 1993, the RAOC was merged with four other army units to form the Royal Logistics Corps.

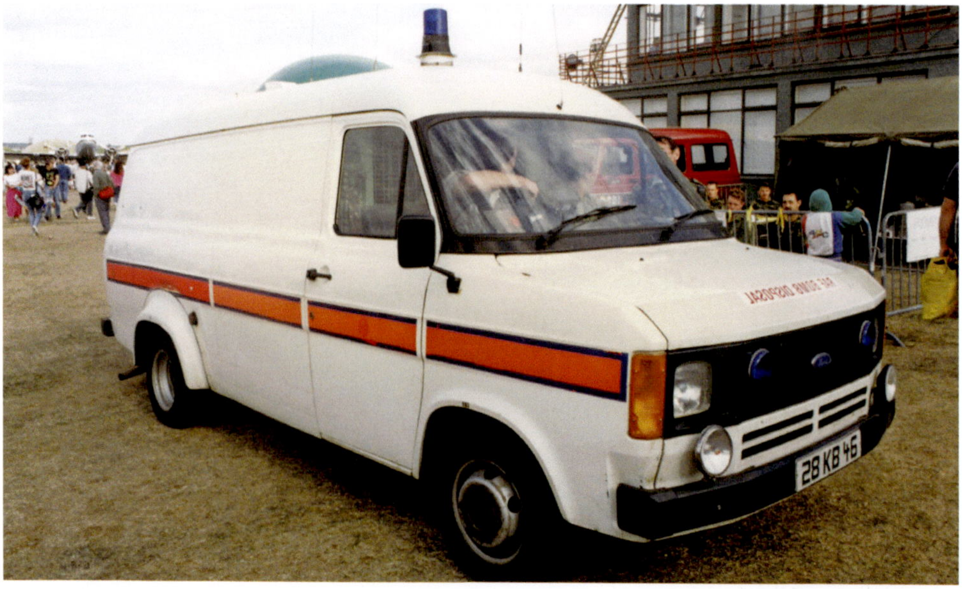

Throughout the 1970s and 1980s, the Royal Air Force staged many Battle of Britain At Home Day air shows at airfields across the UK. The last such show held at RAF Abingdon was in 1991. Seen at RAF Abingdon in the late 1980s was this Ford Transit Mk.2 LWB, EOD team vehicle (dating from the late 1970s/early 1980s), of RAF 5131 (Bomb Disposal) Squadron. With its final base at RAF Wittering in Cambridgeshire, the squadron was disbanded in 2020, its duties transferring to the army.

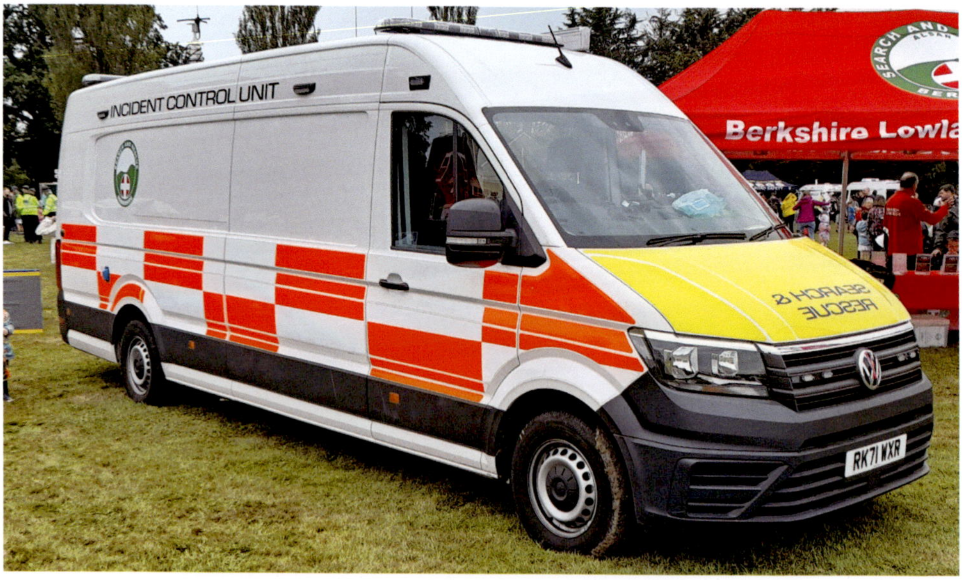

While parts of the UK have mountain rescue teams, other less hilly parts have lowland search and rescue teams, including the Thames Valley. Established in the late 1970s/early 1980s as the South East Berkshire Emergency Volunteers, the team changed its name in 2011 to Berkshire Lowland Search and Rescue. Based near Wokingham, the team is often involved in searches for missing vulnerable people. RK71 WXR (2022) is a VW Crafter used as an ICU.

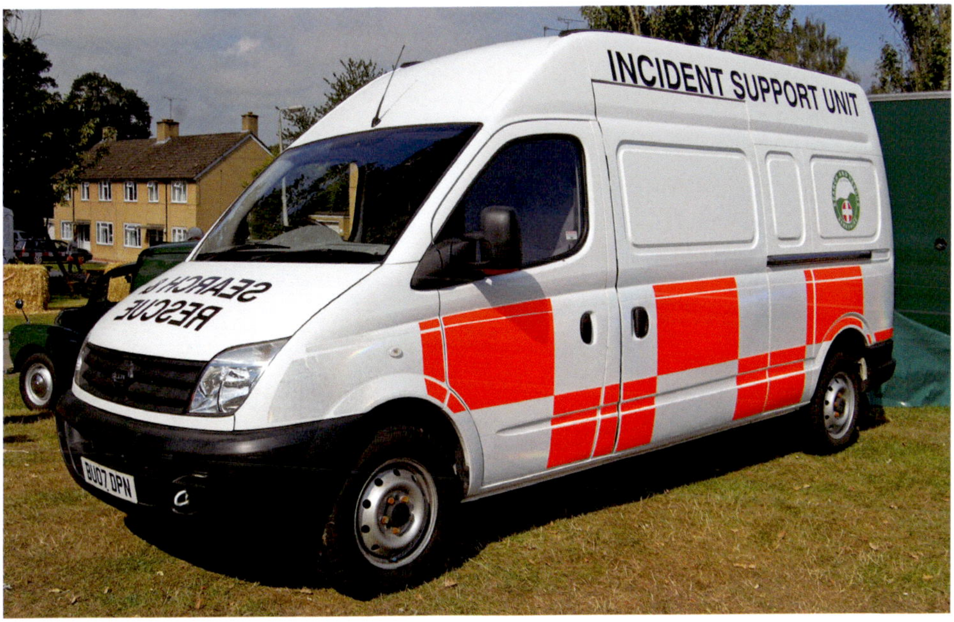

At the time of writing this book (2024), the Berkshire LLSAR team's Incident Support Unit was due for replacement. BU07 DPN (2007) is a LDV Maxus LWB high-roof van. Amongst other items of equipment, the ISU carries four mountain bikes. The team also has a Water Rescue Unit, based on a Renault Master LWB combi van, and also had ICUs based on Mercedes Sprinter and Iveco Daily vans.

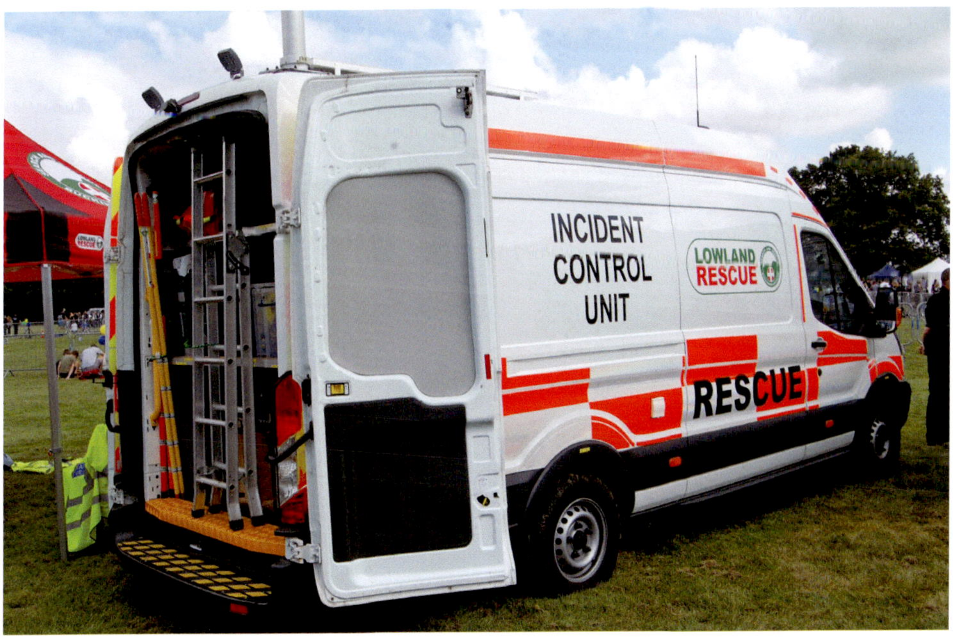

Founded in 1987, Buckinghamshire Search and Rescue is based at Chalfont St Peter, near Gerrards Cross. On display at the Thames Valley Police open day at Sulhamstead in 2023 was their new ICU, a Ford Transit LWB high-roof van.

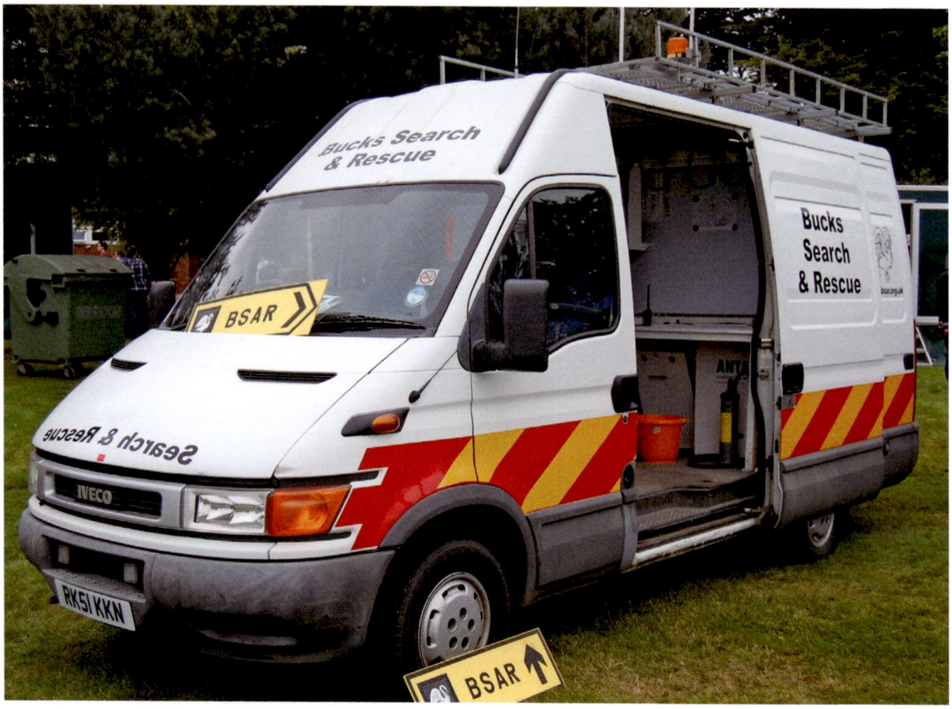

At the 2011 Thames Valley Police open day at Sulhamstead, Buckinghamshire Search and Rescue had their then ICU on display. RK51 KKN (2002) was an Iveco Daily LWB high-roof van.

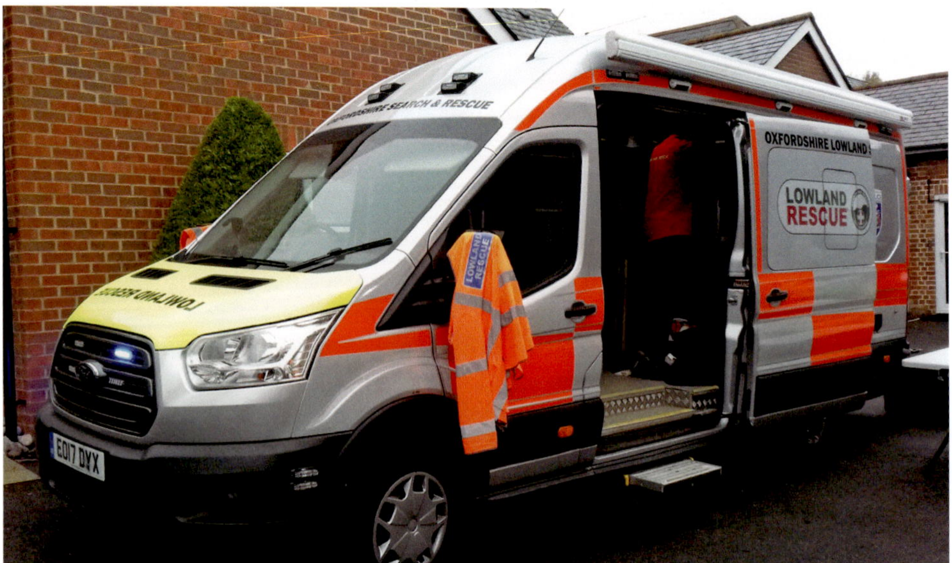

Lowland Rescue Oxfordshire is based at Slade Park Fire Station in the east of Oxford. Seen at an event at Cranford School in Moulsford in south Oxfordshire in 2020 was this Incident Command Unit. EO17 DYX (2017) is a Ford Transit LWB high-roof van; equipment carried includes a drone. The team also has an Incident Support Vehicle, based on a Ford Transit SWB van.

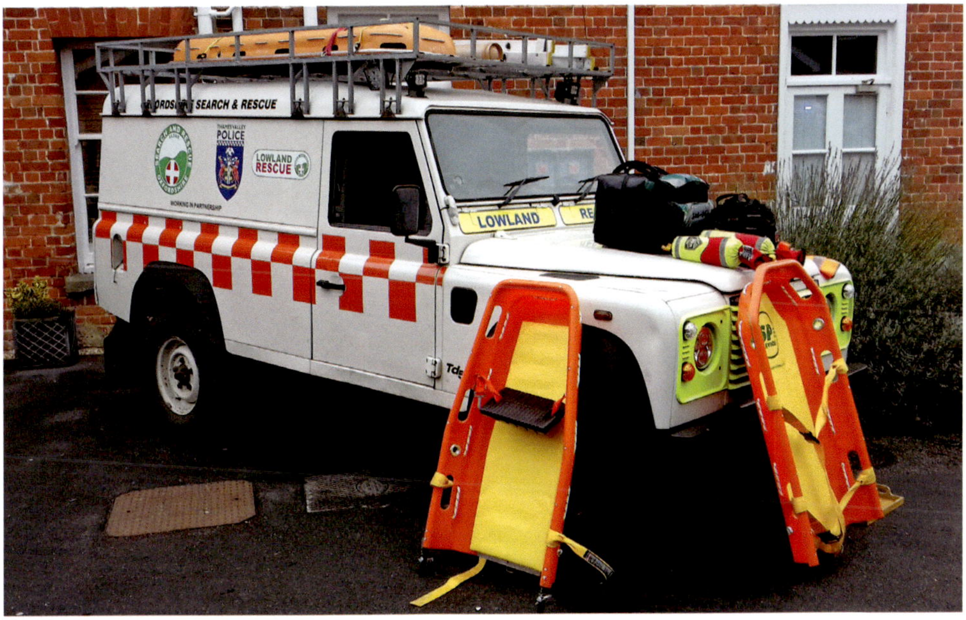

Y728 FFC (2001), a Land Rover Defender 110 Td5 4x4, of Lowland Rescue Oxfordshire, seen at the same event as the ICU. Equipment carried included two stretchers, medical kit, throw lines and a short extension ladder. This vehicle was replaced by a new Toyota Hi-Lux double cab 4x4 in 2021. Established in 2008 as Isis Search and Rescue, the team name changed to Oxfordshire Lowland Search and Rescue, before changing again to its current title.

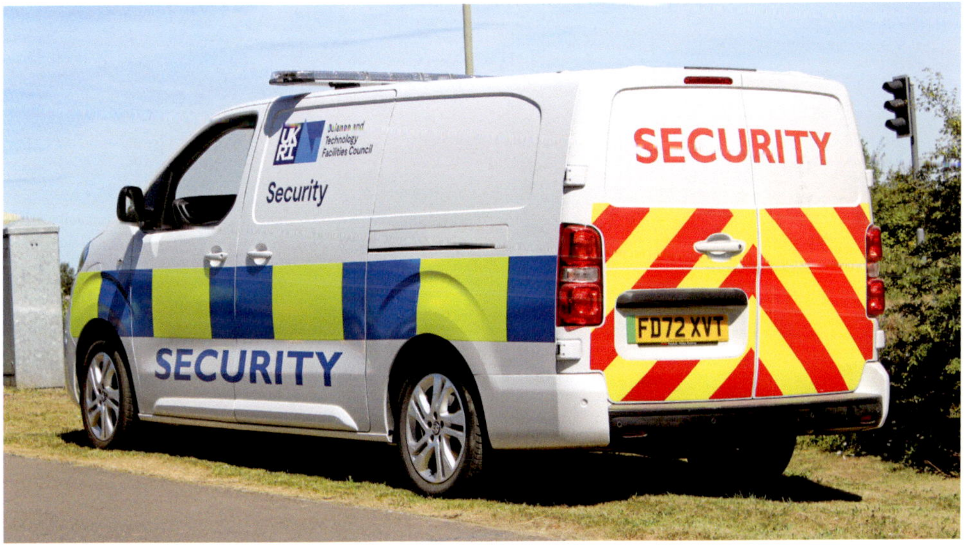

In 1957, land south of AERE Harwell became the site of the Rutherford Appleton Laboratory, which has developed into one of the largest, most advanced, multi-disciplinary science and engineering research centres in Europe. The security vehicle fleet is now all electric and two Vauxhall Vivaro E electric vans were purchased in 2022. Seen on the day of the Harwell and Rutherford open day in June 2024, the crew of FD72 XVT were assisting with traffic management near the junction of the A34 and the A4185 at Chilton.

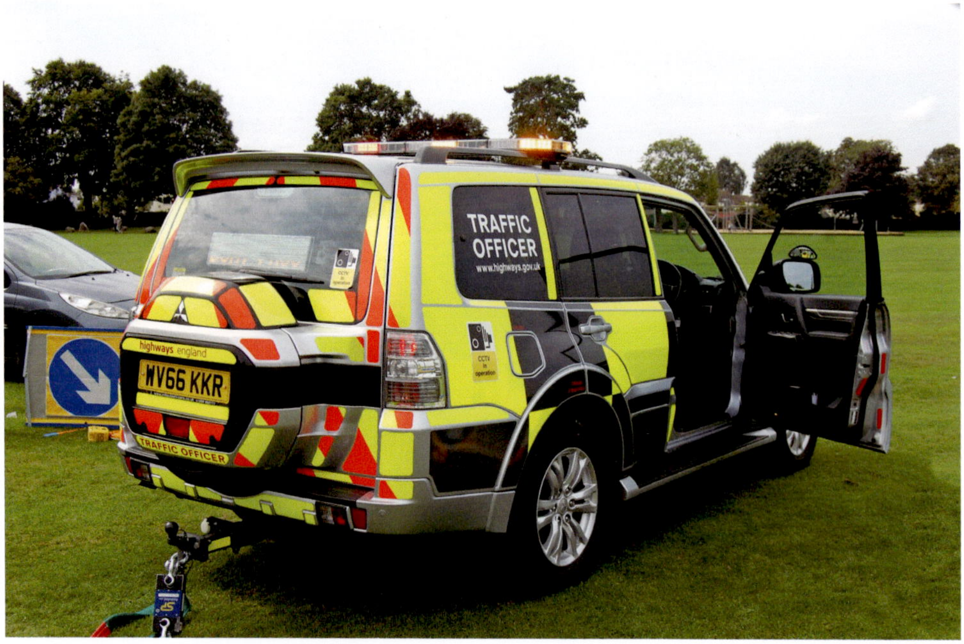

On display at an Emergency Services event in Didcot in 2017 was WV66 KKR, an almost brand-new Mitsubishi Shogun 4x4 Traffic Officer Vehicle. Set up with towing straps attached and digital sign scrolling through messages, this TOV was then part of the Highways England fleet.

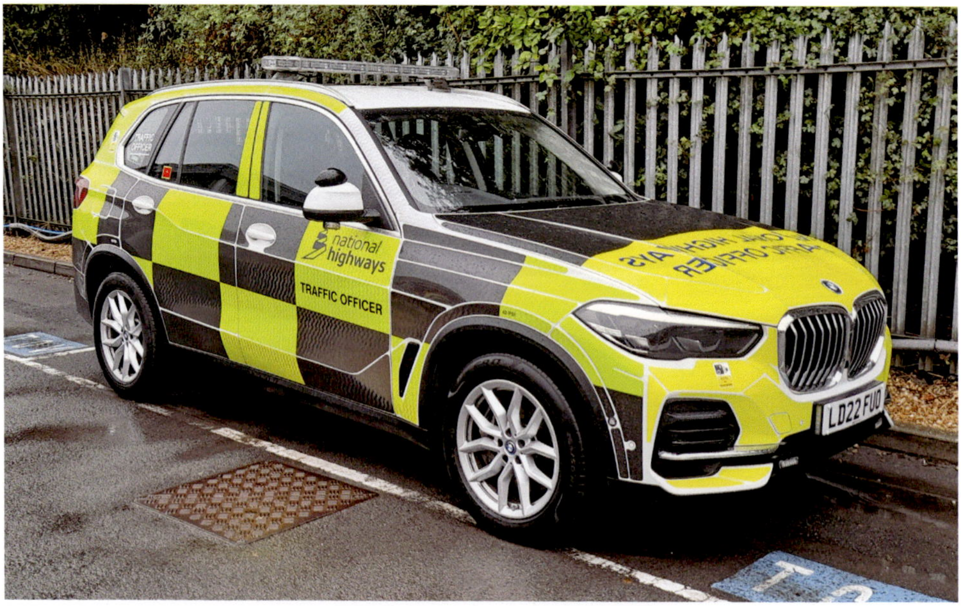

National Highways has three Traffic Officer Out-Stations in the Thames Valley, at Bray and Chieveley (Berkshire) and Milton Common (Oxfordshire). One of the Traffic Officer Vehicles at the Chieveley Out-Station, north of Newbury, covering the M4, is LD22 FUO (2022), a BMW X5 Xdrive 4x4 hybrid.

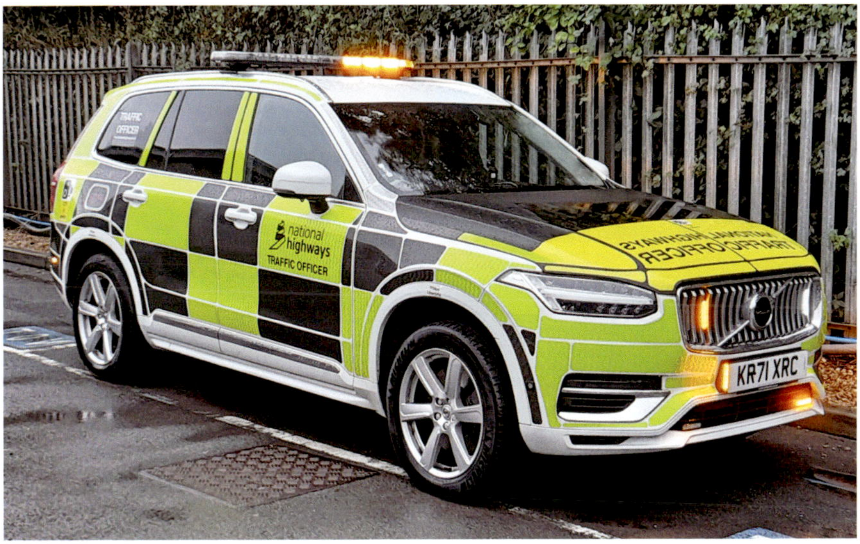

Since 2021, National Highways has purchased over 300 Plug-in Hybrid Electric Vehicles, many for its Traffic Officers. One of them is this Volvo XC90 4x4 Recharge T8 Traffic Officer Vehicle based at Chieveley. Equipment carried includes twenty traffic cones, six signs, flashing lights, crowbar, broom, shovel and an AED.

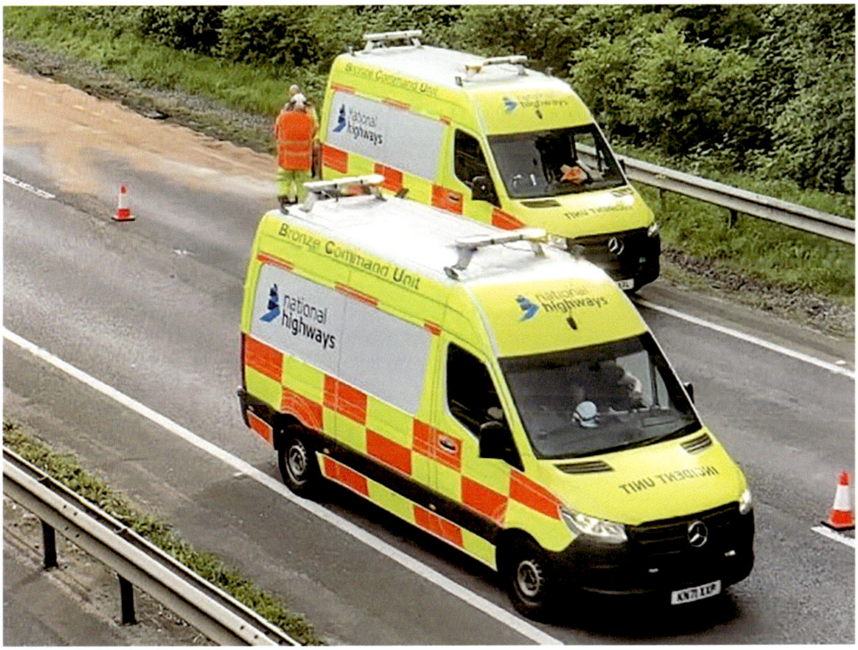

One of the busiest roads in southern England is the A34 dual carriageway between the M4 and the M40, which often experiences congestion, incidents and delays. During the evening rush hour on 16 May 2024, a diesel spill on the northbound carriageway at Chilton in Oxfordshire was attended to by TVP, Oxfordshire F&RS, National Highways Traffic Officers and two National Highways Incident Units (Mercedes Sprinter 315 CDi vans). The inside lane needed resurfacing following the clean-up.

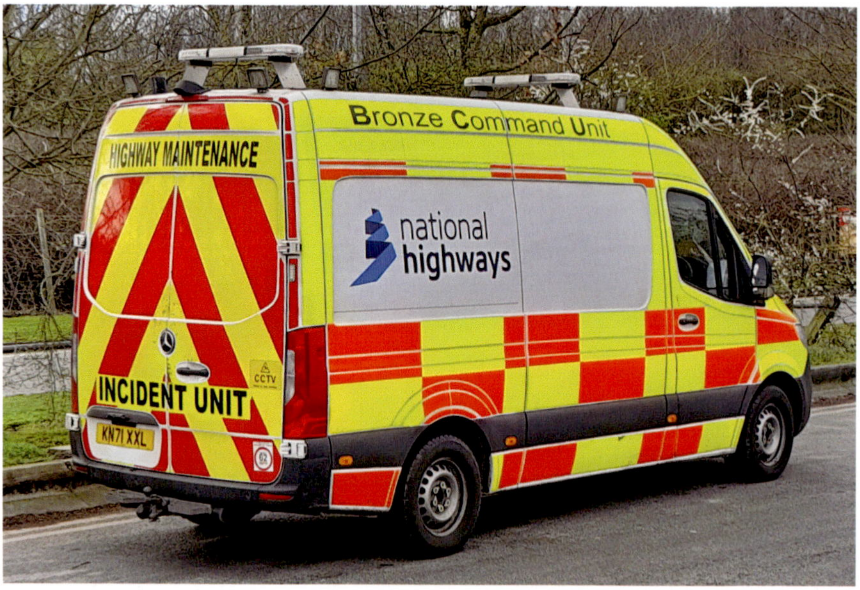

Seen parked near Milton Interchange in Oxfordshire, roughly halfway between the M4 and the M40, is KN71 XXL (2021), one of the National Highways' Mercedes Sprinter 315 CDi, Incident Units, which perform an 'Attend and Assess' role to determine any repair work and resources required following an incident. A command structure of Operational (Bronze), Tactical (Silver) and Strategic (Gold) is used for large-scale, multi-agency incidents by the emergency services and other responders.

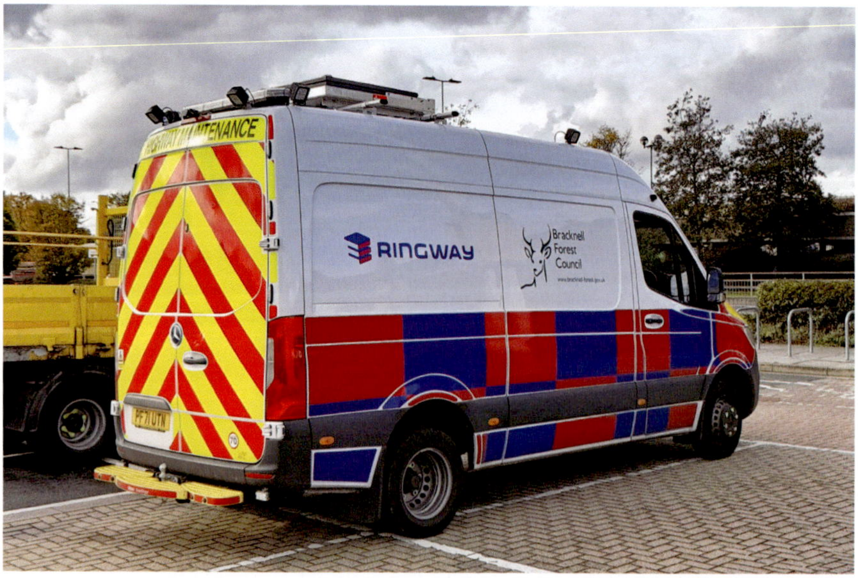

With its head office in West Sussex, Ringway manages over 43,000 km (over 27,000 miles) of roads in the UK, working in partnership with local authorities, including Bracknell Forest Council in Berkshire. PF71 UTN (2022) is a Mercedes Sprinter 515 CDi, Highways Maintenance/ Incident Unit, seen in Bracknell when almost new. Mounted on the roof is a folding digital warning sign.

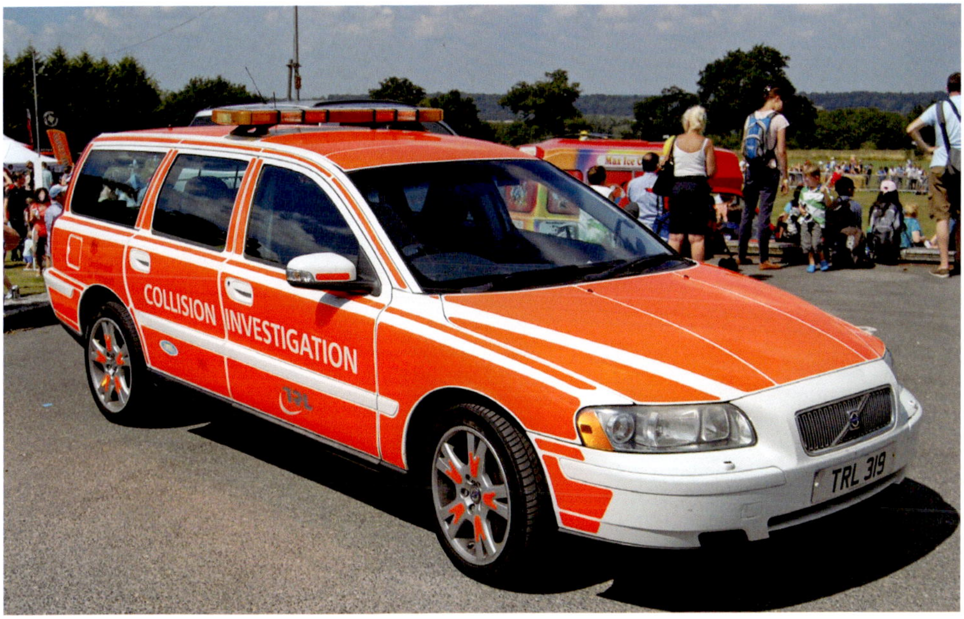

An eye-catching, non-Battenberg, highly visible, almost all-over orange livery was applied to this Volvo V70 estate car used by TRL (Transport Research Laboratory) as a Collision Investigation Unit. TRL, located in Crowthorne (Berkshire), is a wholly owned subsidiary of the Transport Research Foundation. Previously, TRL used a Mercedes E-Class estate car as a CIU. TRL 319 was almost brand new when displayed at the 2015, TVP, Sulhamstead open day.

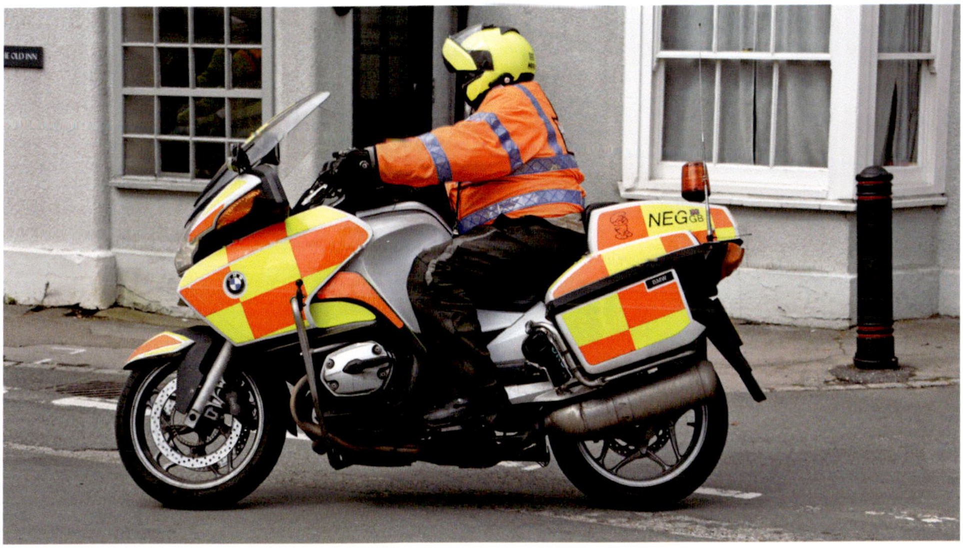

A National Escort Group (NEG – an organisation providing trained marshals for sporting events) BMW motorcycle escorting the men's Tour of Britain cycle race through Brill in Buckinghamshire in September 2017. The Thames Valley area has hosted several stages of both the men's and women's Tour of Britain cycle races, featuring well-known cyclists such as Mark Cavendish from the Isle of Man, Geraint Thomas and Elynor Bäckstedt from Wales and local rider Katie Scott from Oxford.

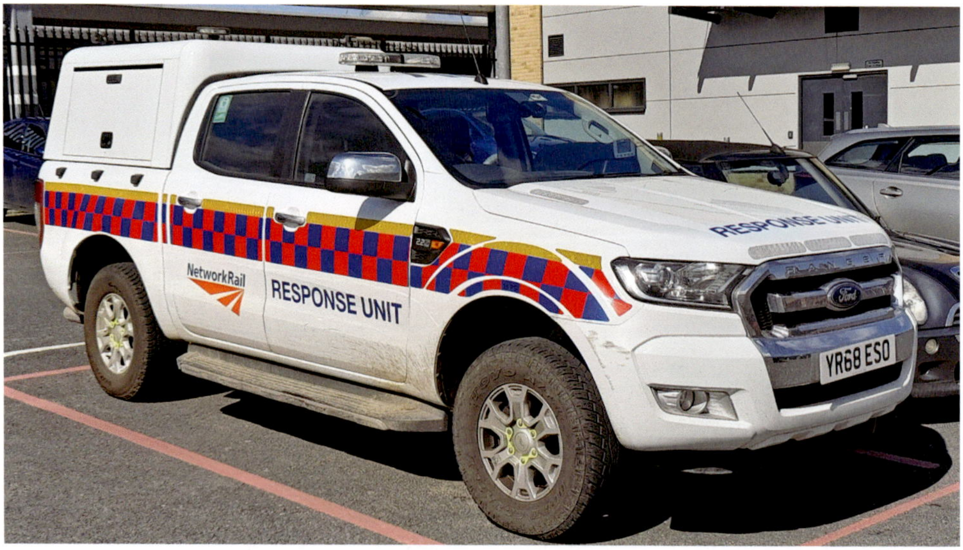

YR68 ESO (2018), a Ford Ranger 4x4 2.2l Network Rail Response Unit, seen in front of Oxford railway station in April 2023. Network Rail owns and maintains the majority of the railway infrastructure in Great Britain. Using a fleet of four-wheel-drive vehicles and vans, Network Rail has Mobile Operations Managers who respond to situations affecting the railways and if required act as Rail Incident Officers.

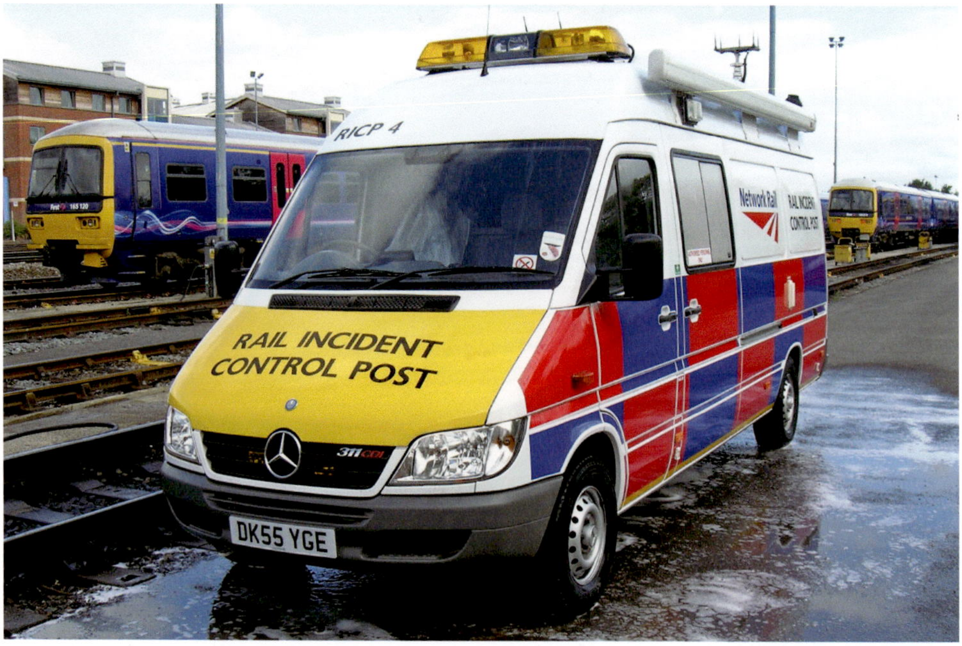

DK55 YGE (2005), RICP 4, a Mercedes Sprinter 311 CDi LWB van. Initially based at Didcot, this Rail Incident Control Post had been relocated to Oxford when photographed in 2008. At the 2024 Emergency Services Show, a new Rail Incident Command Vehicle, based on a Ford Transit LWB van, was displayed. (Photo: Richard Roberts – N.B. The photographer was trained and authorised to work track-side)

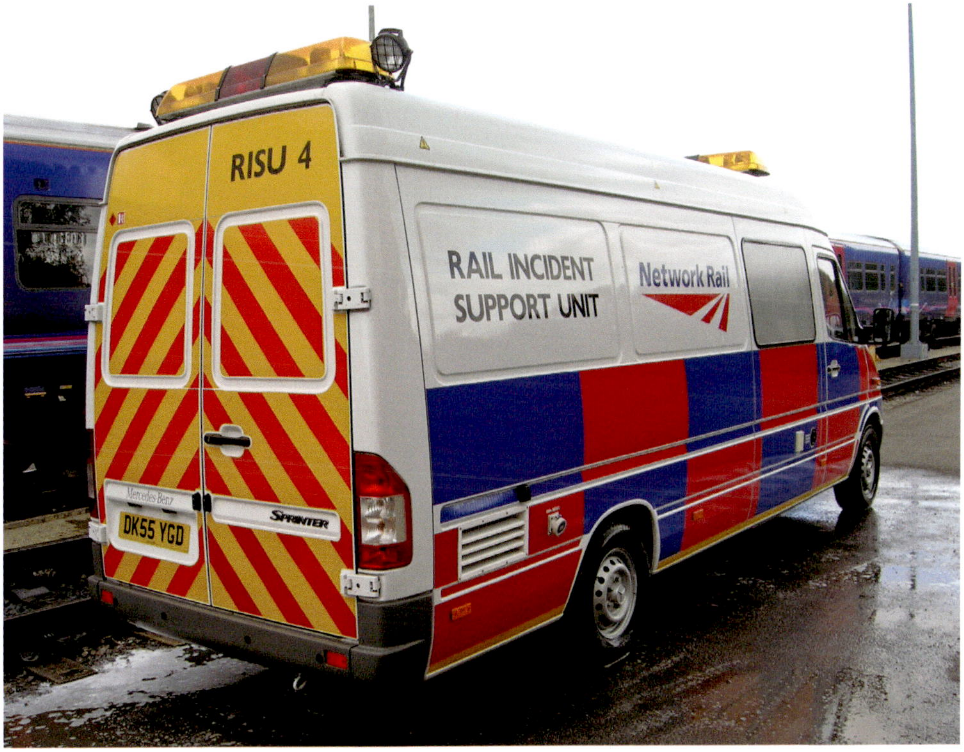

DK55 YGD (2005), RISU 4, another Mercedes Sprinter 311 CDi LWB van. Also at Oxford, having been at Didcot previously, was this Rail Incident Support Unit. These vehicles were based in five pairs around England and Scotland. (Photo: Richard Roberts – N.B. The photographer was trained and authorised to work track-side)

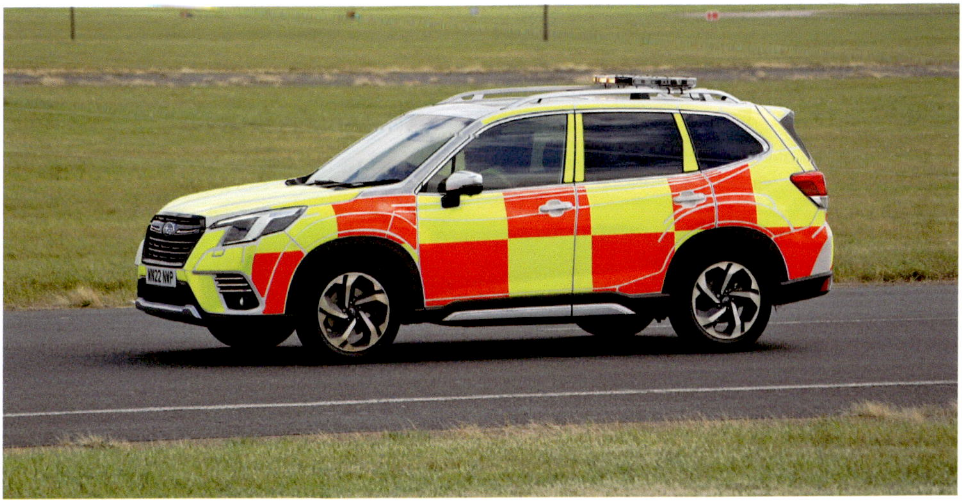

One of the vehicles used in support of airfield operations at RAF Benson in Oxfordshire is this hybrid Subaru Forester 4x4 SUV. This vehicle is used to undertake airside safety and bird control roles. The yellow and orange Battenberg markings contrast with the predominately green background, allowing the vehicle to be visible across the airfield.

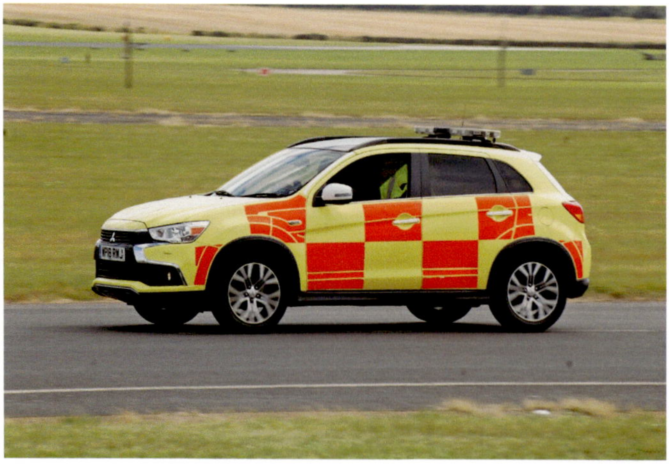

Another of the vehicles used in support of airfield operations at RAF Benson is this Mitsubishi ASX crossover-style car. This vehicle is used to undertake airside safety and wildlife hazard management roles. Both vehicles were seen during the RAF Benson Families Day in August 2024. Just after the photos were taken, a six-vehicle RTC occurred on the A4074 south of the airfield.

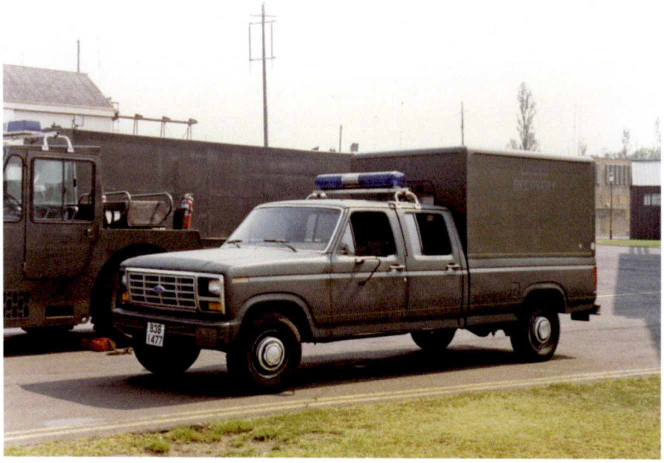

This 1983 Ford F-350, LWB, double cab 4x4, fitted with a box body, was one of three USAF Crash Recovery vehicles seen during the air show at RAF Upper Heyford, located in the north of Oxfordshire, in 1991. The black Crash Recovery lettering is barely visible against the matt green colour. Parked adjacent to the vehicle is a large aircraft towing tug, which was also fitted with a blue light-bar.

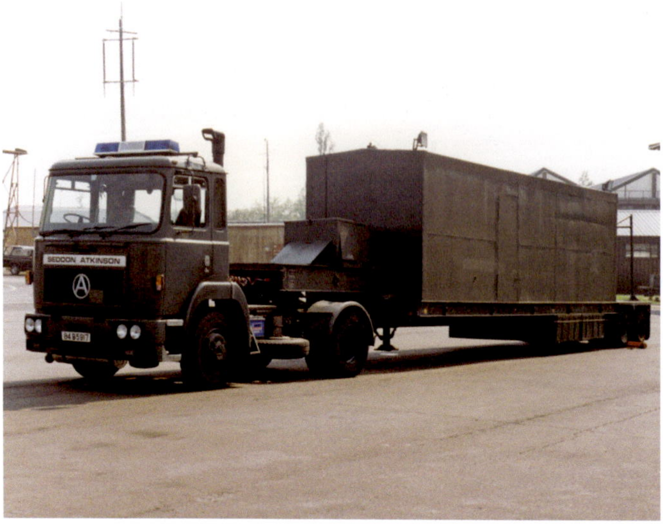

Towing a Crash Recovery articulated trailer was this 1984, British-built Seddon Atkinson 401 tractor unit. The USAF also used British-built Bedford CF and Freight Rover Sherpa vehicles. Having been the base for F-111 multi-role combat aircraft during the 1970s and 1980s, the last aircraft left Upper Heyford in 1993 and the airfield was handed back to the MoD in 1994. The airfield is now used for business, housing and police specialist training.

Chapter 4
Police Forces

The three counties of Berkshire, Buckinghamshire and Oxfordshire are covered by one Home Office territorial police force, the Thames Valley Police (TVP). It is the largest non-metropolitan police force in England, covering an area of 5,742 square kilometres (2,218 square miles). The population of just over 2.4 million people lives in a diverse range of communities in a mix of locations ranging from large urban areas, new towns, historic market towns, to rural villages, tiny hamlets, isolated farms and country houses.

The force was formed on 1 April 1968 as the Thames Valley Constabulary, with the amalgamation of the Berkshire, Buckinghamshire, Oxfordshire, Oxford City and Reading Borough police forces. The force's name was changed to the current title in 1971.

With its headquarters on two sites in Kidlington (Oxfordshire), the force was divided into eleven Local Policing Areas, based on one or more local authority areas, but starting in April 2024, this is changing to a new five Local Command Area structure, based on Berkshire East, Berkshire West, Buckinghamshire, Milton Keynes and Oxfordshire.

There are two control rooms, at Abingdon (Oxfordshire) and Milton Keynes (Buckinghamshire). The main training centre (including firearms and dog training) is located at Sulhamstead (Berkshire), with public order training carried out at Upper Heyford (Oxfordshire) and driver training based at Banbury (Oxfordshire). Vehicle workshops are located at Bicester (Oxfordshire) and Sulhamstead. A new forensics centre is due to open in 2025, adjacent to the Roads Policing Unit and vehicle workshops in Bicester.

A Joint Operations Unit with the Hampshire and Isle of Wight Constabulary includes the Roads Policing Unit with bases at Abingdon and Bicester (Oxfordshire); Three Mile Cross (Reading, Berkshire); Amersham, Milton Keynes and Taplow (Buckinghamshire, which is also the base for the force's Protection Group, an armed unit which is in addition to the TVP's Armed Response Vehicles). The force's Mounted Section is based at Milton Keynes and has seven horses. A National Police Air Service helicopter is based at RAF Benson (Oxfordshire).

In addition to the TVP, five non-Home Office, non-territorial police forces operate within the Thames Valley area, namely British Transport Police, Civil Nuclear Constabulary, Ministry of Defence Police, Royal Air Force Police and Royal Military Police. Furthermore, the Metropolitan Police protects Windsor Castle.

THAMES VALLEY POLICE

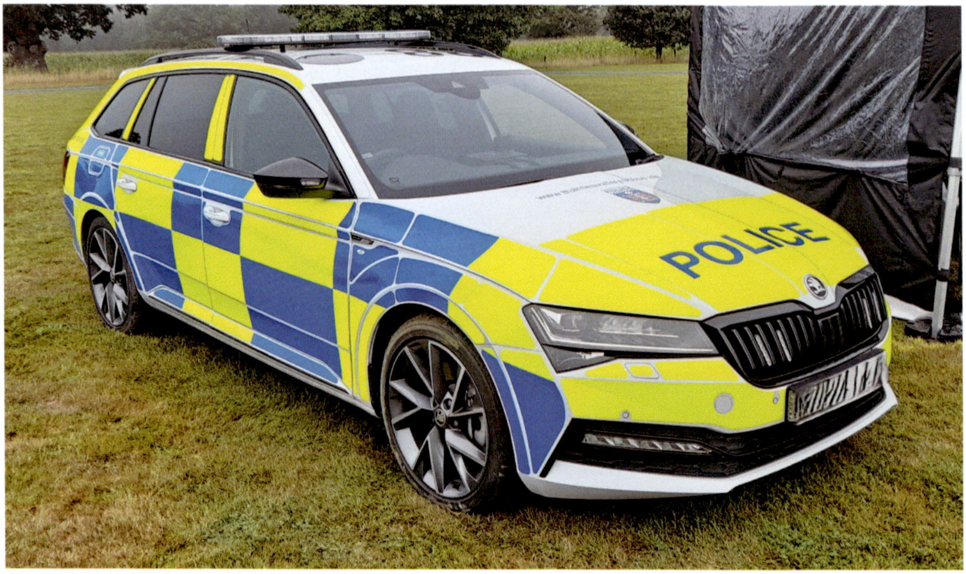

Two of the newest vehicles on display at the 2024 annual Thames Valley Police open day at the Sulhamstead Training Centre in Berkshire were a pair of new driver training vehicles. The Skoda Superb 2.0-litre estate cars are a new type of vehicle in the TVP fleet. Driver Training is based at Banbury Police Station in Oxfordshire.

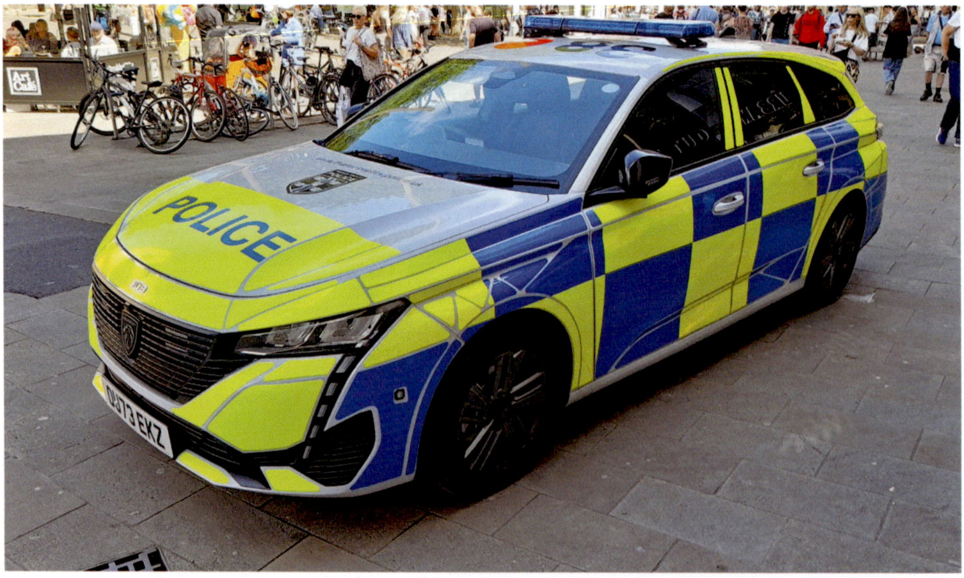

Seen in a very busy Oxford city centre, with Bonn Square and Queen Street in the background, during the afternoon of 16 August 2024 was this Peugeot 308 Active HDI 1.5-litre diesel estate, OU73 EKZ (2023). It was one of the first vehicles to display the new TVP badge, launched in the summer of 2024. This vehicle has full Battenberg markings on the sides but no police lettering on the doors.

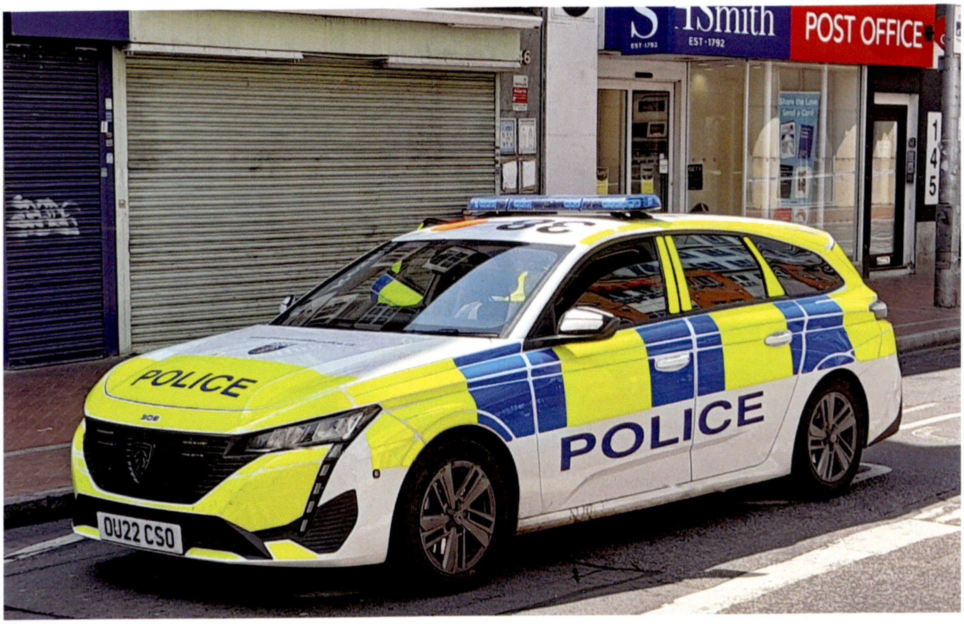

Starting in 2020, the Peugeot 308 estate car has been used in the role of Beat Car/Immediate Response Vehicle across TVP. OU22 CSO (2022) is a Peugeot 308 Active HDI 1.5-litre diesel estate, which was at the cordon for a road closure during a Make Pumps Ten fire in Friar Street, Reading, in May 2023. This vehicle has half Battenberg markings on the sides and police lettering on the doors.

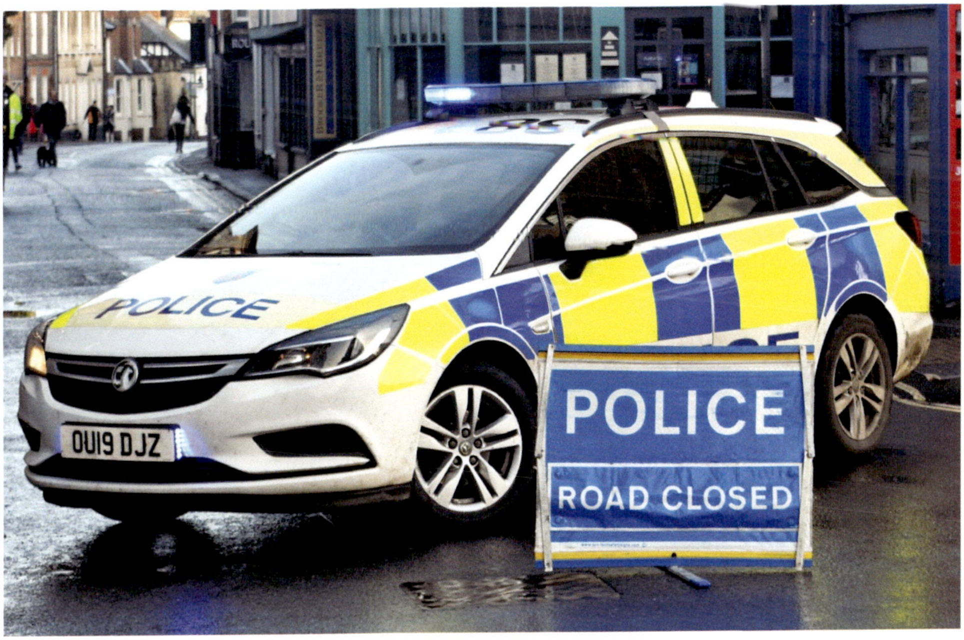

OU19 DJZ (2019) is a Vauxhall Astra Mk.7 1.6-litre diesel estate, which was in use at a road closure in High Street, Wallingford. This was due to a narrowboat colliding with the north side of Wallingford Bridge over the River Thames on the day after Boxing Day in December 2022.

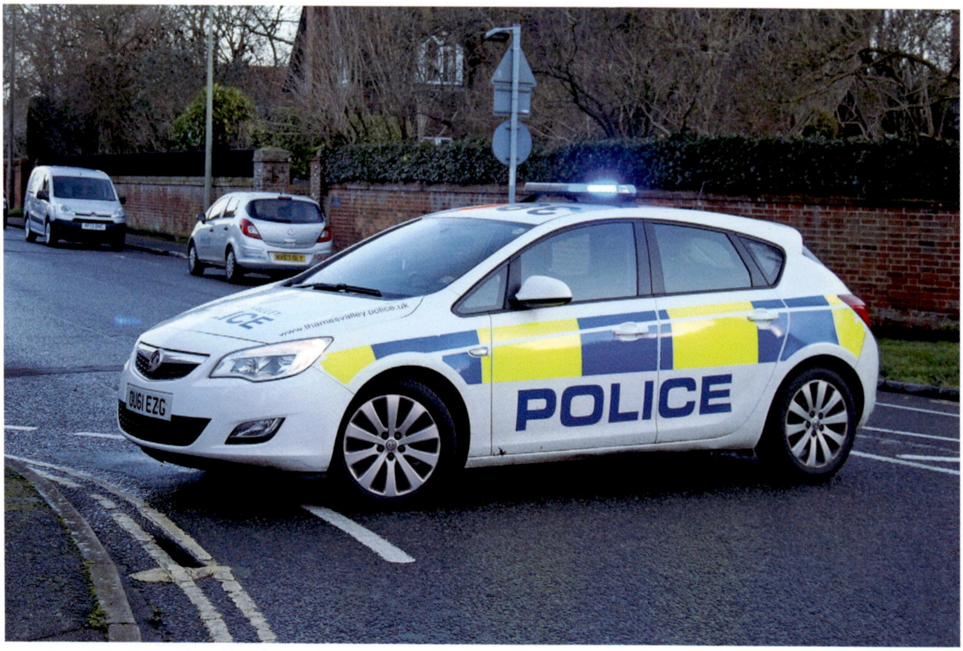

TVP has used the Vauxhall Astra, mainly the hatchback version, since the Mk.2 was launched in the mid-1980s. OU61 EZG (2012) is a Vauxhall Astra Mk.6 hatchback in use at a road closure in Crowmarsh due to a large fire which almost completely destroyed the offices of the South Oxfordshire District Council in January 2015.

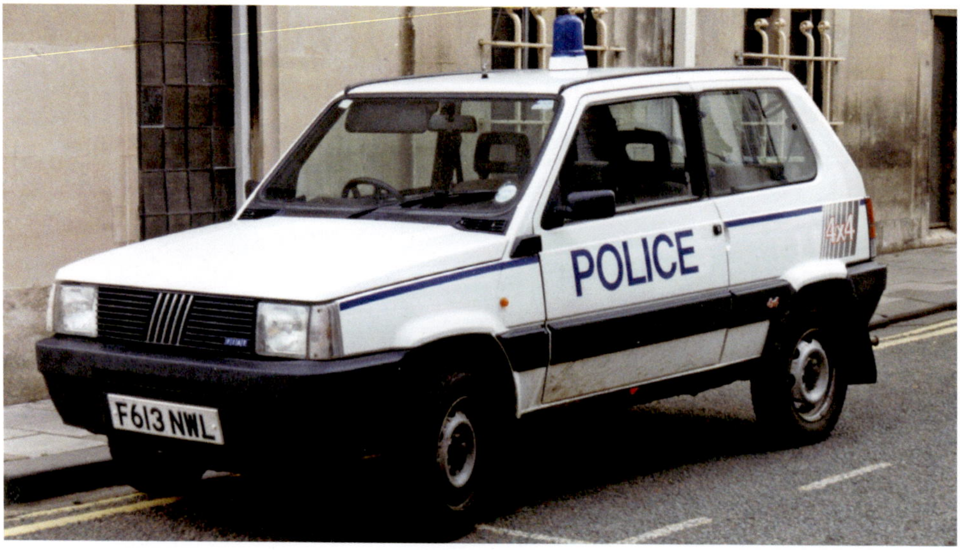

Although some were used as police vehicles in their native Italy, an unusual choice for a beat ('Panda') car in the UK was the appropriately named Fiat Panda. Photographed in the early 1990s while parked outside the town hall in Henley-on-Thames (Oxfordshire), opposite the former police station, was F613 NWL, a 1989 Mk.1, 1-litre petrol engine, 4x4 version. The drive-train and four-wheel-drive system were made in Austria by Steyr-Daimler-Puch. (Photo: Colin Dunford)

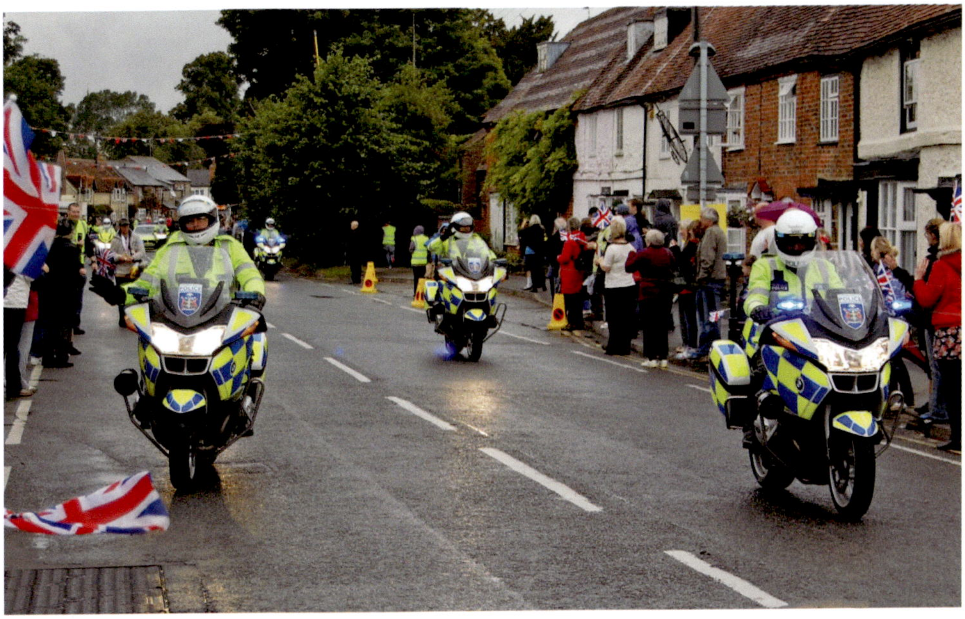

10 July 2012 was day 53 of the Olympic Torch relay through the UK, with the torch being carried from Oxford to Reading. Ahead of the Olympic Torch, six TVP roads policing BMW RT motorcycles have just crossed the River Thames over Wallingford Bridge and have entered the village of Crowmarsh on their way to Henley before crossing into Berkshire.

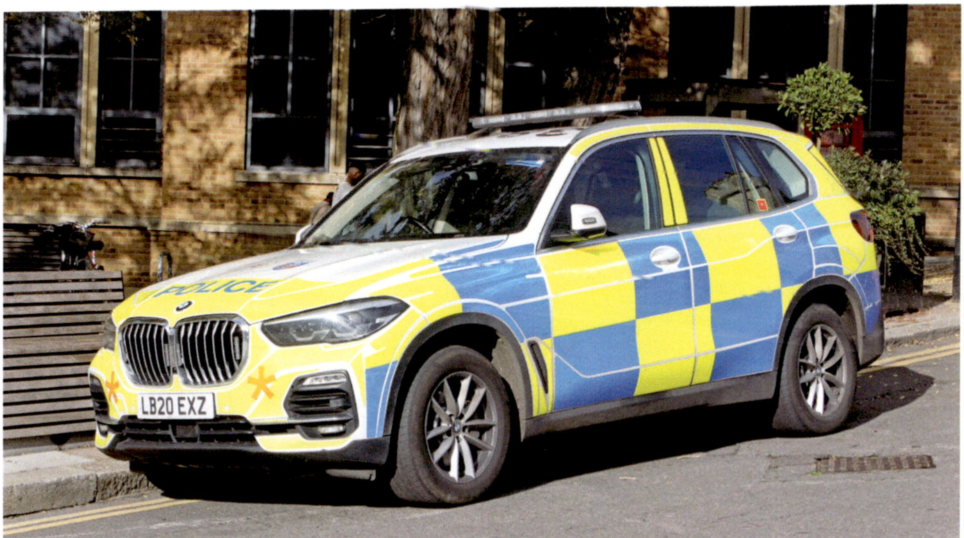

Thames Valley Police provides an armed escort to military personnel participating in the Changing of the Guard parade from Victoria Barracks to Windsor Castle and back. Following a parade in October 2023, this TVP Armed Response Vehicle (ARV), LB20 EXZ (2020), a BMW X5 4x4, was parked in St Alban's Street. The small red sticker on the rear door window indicates to other emergency services that the vehicle is fitted with two batteries, rather than just the one, in case it is involved in a collision. (Photo: Gethin Roberts)

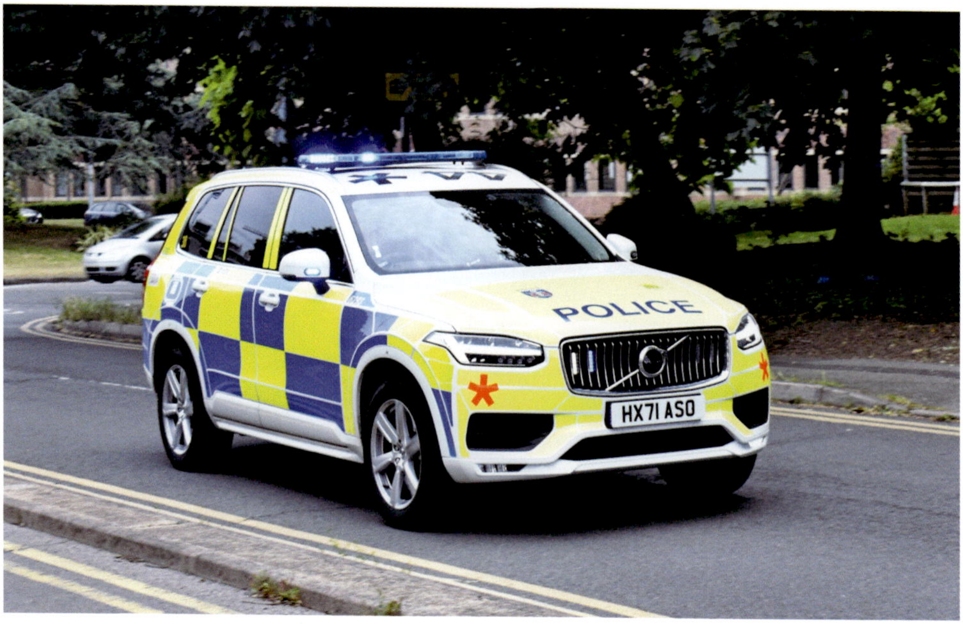

An example of a Joint Operations Unit vehicle is this Hampshire and Isle of Wight Constabulary Volvo XC90 hybrid AWD, ARV. Approaching Maidenhead Fire Station during the open day in 2022 was HX71 ASO (2021). Visible on the roof above the driver's door is the black star (or asterisk, or snowflake) symbol, indicating to the crew of a police helicopter or drone operator that it is an ARV; the force identifying number for the HIOW Constabulary is 44.

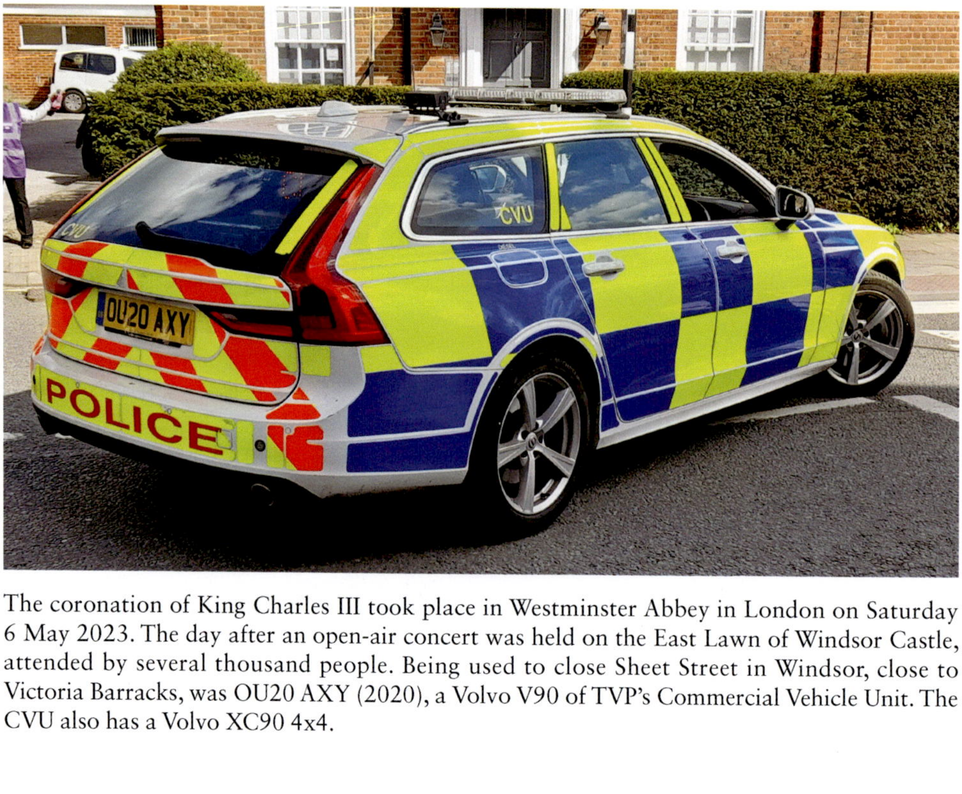

The coronation of King Charles III took place in Westminster Abbey in London on Saturday 6 May 2023. The day after an open-air concert was held on the East Lawn of Windsor Castle, attended by several thousand people. Being used to close Sheet Street in Windsor, close to Victoria Barracks, was OU20 AXY (2020), a Volvo V90 of TVP's Commercial Vehicle Unit. The CVU also has a Volvo XC90 4x4.

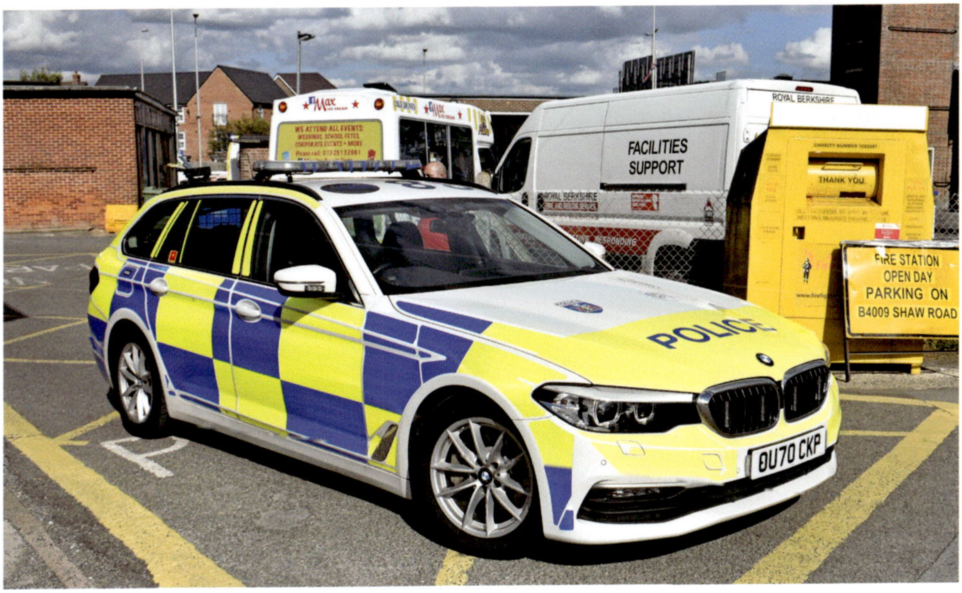

At the end of an open day in August 2022, a very patient but no doubt relieved Roads Policing Officer exits the drill yard of Newbury Fire Station, having let countless children sit in his car and operate the lights and siren. OU70 CKP (2020) is a BMW 530d Touring of TVP's Roads Policing Unit. Visible on the roof above the driver's door is the black circle symbol, indicating to the crew of a police helicopter or drone operator that it is an incident response or roads policing vehicle; the force identifying number for TVP is 38.

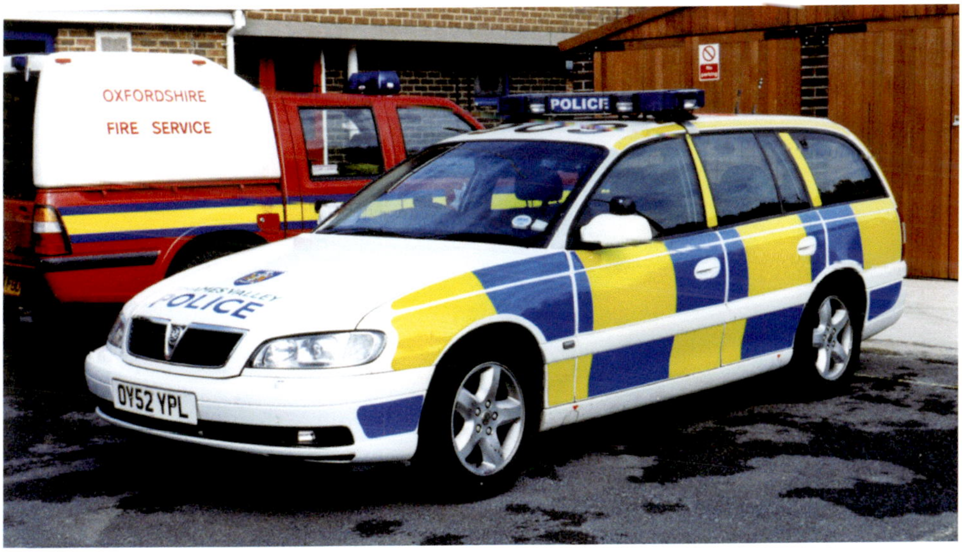

Seen on a visit to Abingdon Fire Station in the mid-2000s was this Vauxhall Omega V6 estate traffic car. OY52 YPL (2002) was based at the nearby Abingdon Police Station, from which it could easily access the A34 Winchester to Salford trunk road. In 1989, a pile-up involving thirty-one vehicles occurred on the northbound carriageway near Drayton, south of Abingdon, with smoke from stubble burning drifting across the dual carriageway. This led to legislation to control stubble burning in England and Wales in 1993.

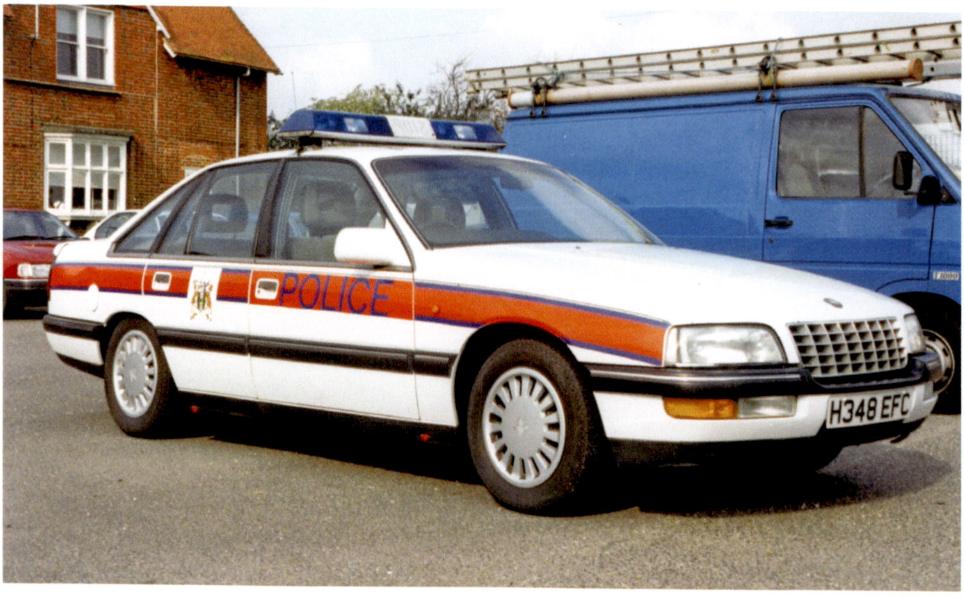

The Vauxhall Senator 3.0-litre 24v was considered by many police officers to have been the best traffic car of the late 1980s/early 1990s. The executive saloon car, built in Germany by Opel, was a popular choice with police forces across the UK and TVP used both the Mk.1 and the restyled Mk.2. Photographed in the early 1990s, outside Gerrard's Cross Police Station in Buckinghamshire, was H348 EFC, a Mk.2 version dating from 1990. Another TVP Senator (L345 KUD) took part in the trial of the Battenberg livery in the mid-1990s.

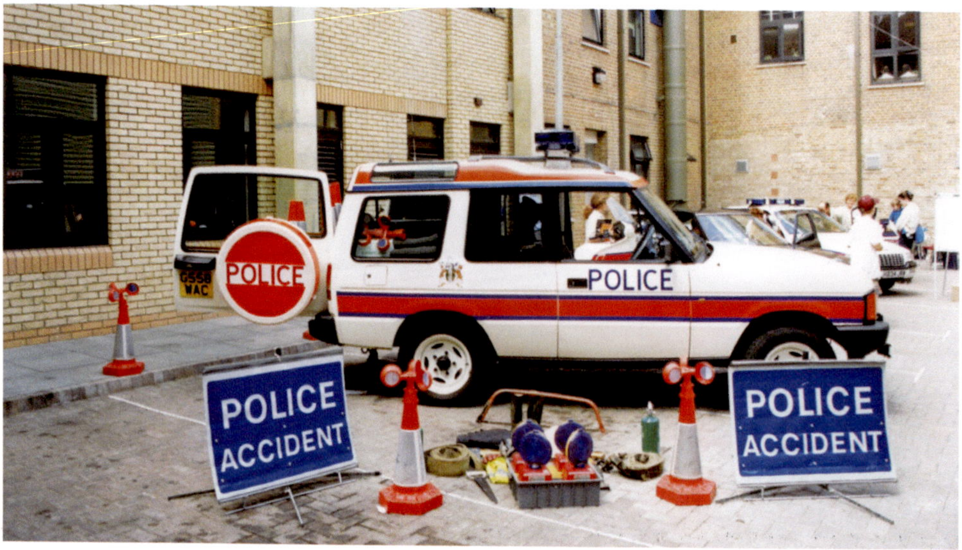

In the early 1990s, St Aldate's Police Station in the centre of Oxford was refurbished and an open day was held in July 1991. On display in the inner courtyard was one of TVP's first Land Rover Discovery Mk.1 Accident Units. G558 WAC and three other TVP Discoveries were registered in Warwickshire in 1990, so may have been supplied directly by Land Rover. Fitted with a light-mast and carrying twenty-four cones, several warning signs and numerous other items of equipment, call-sign Tango Charlie Nine Nine was based at Bicester.

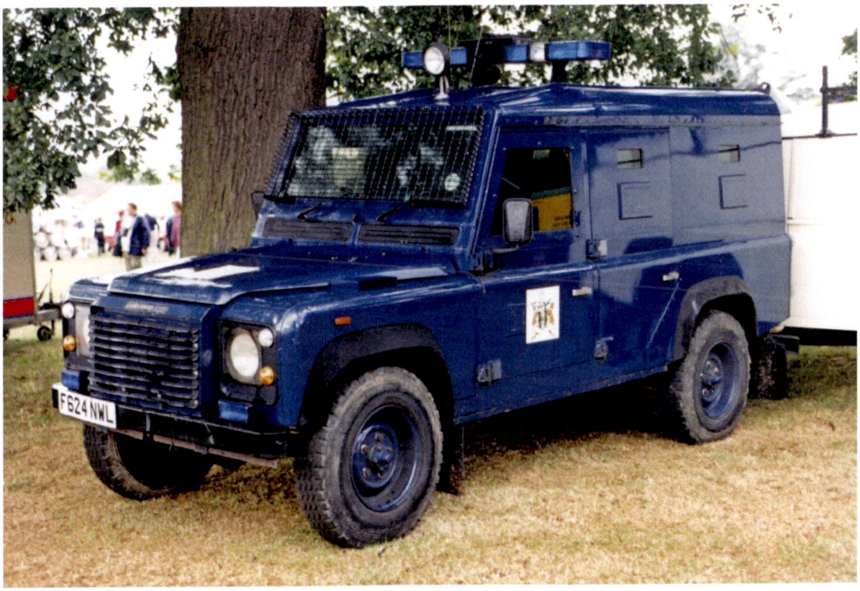

Following a tragic mass casualty shooting incident in Hungerford in Berkshire in August 1987 in which seventeen people (including the gunman) died, one of the findings of a report was that Thames Valley Police should have two armoured vehicles. In 1989, two Land Rover 110 V8 4x4 vans were armoured by a specialist firm for use by the force's firearms officers and were based at the HQ in Kidlington. F624 NWL was on display at an emergency services event in Reading in 1995; the other vehicle was registered F614 NWL.

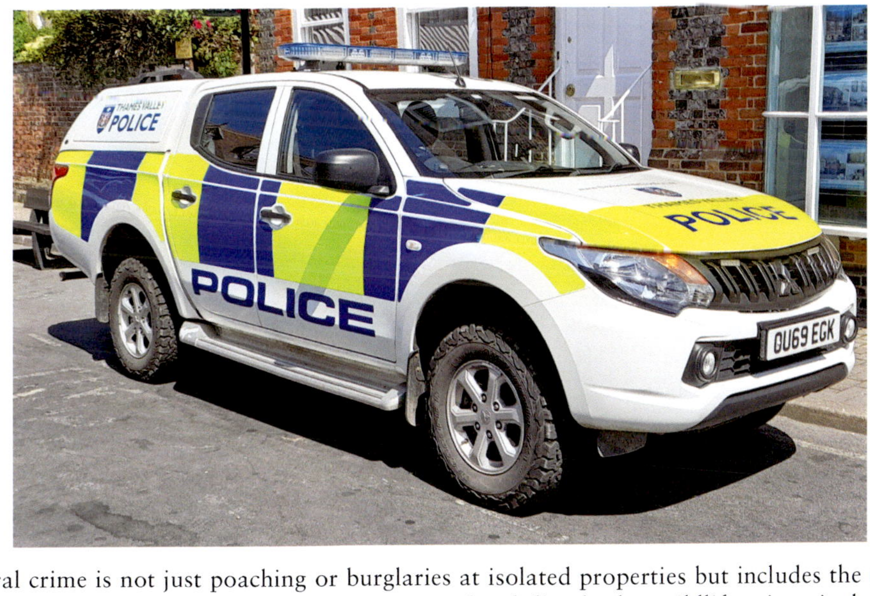

Rural crime is not just poaching or burglaries at isolated properties but includes the theft of expensive farm machinery, GPS systems and red diesel, plus wildlife crime, including hare coursing (sometimes filmed or live streamed for gambling), and the illegal dumping of waste, sometimes hazardous, known as fly-tipping. To patrol rural areas, TVP has several Mitsubishi L200 and Ford Ranger 4x4s. OU69 EGK (2019), a Mitsubishi L200 4x4 2.4d, was seen in Wantage in Oxfordshire in June 2023.

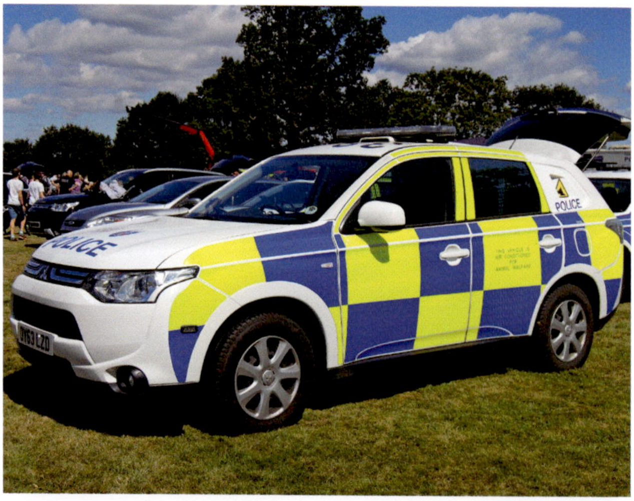

Having used Ford Escort and Vauxhall Astra vans as Dog Units for many years, followed by Vauxhall Zafira MPVs, TVP purchased the third generation Mitsubishi Outlander crossover SUV in the early 2010s. This example was taking part in an open day at TVP's Training School at Sulhamstead. The lettering on the side states 'This Vehicle Is Air Conditioned For Animal Welfare'. Ford Mondeo estate cars, both marked and unmarked, are now used as Dog Units.

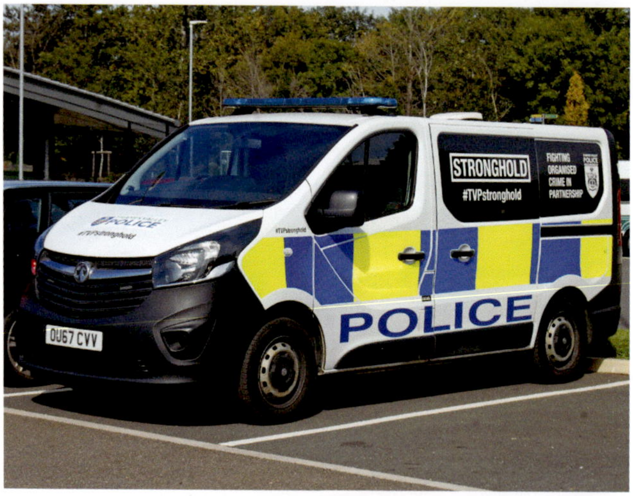

TVP has a large fleet of British-built Vauxhall Vivaro combi-type vans with a cell cage in the rear. OU67 CVV (2017) was seen at the 2023 open day at the Blue Light Hub at West Ashland in Milton Keynes, Buckinghamshire. This vehicle is one of several vans across the Thames Valley promoting the Stronghold initiative, aimed at fighting organised crime.

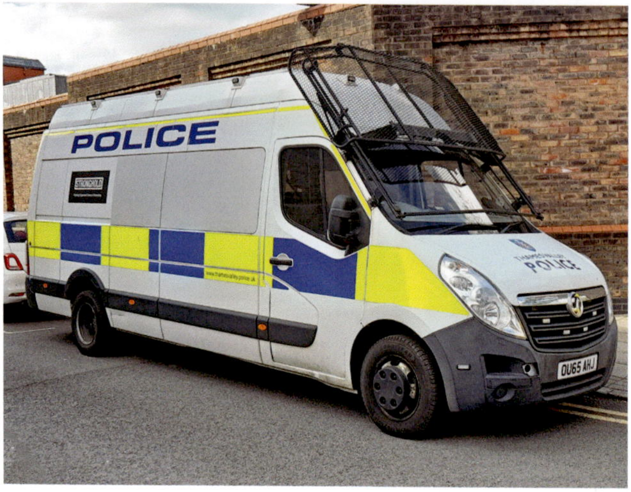

Having used Ford Transit vans for many years and some Freight Rover Sherpa high-roof vans, Vauxhall Movano LWB high-roof vans were purchased as personnel carriers/public order vehicles. OU65 AHJ (2015) was seen in Windsor the day after the coronation of King Charles III. Another Vauxhall Movano, without a grille but fitted with an awning, was used as a Search Team vehicle. Mercedes Sprinter vans are also used. TVP deployed officers to support other forces during civil disturbances in the summer of 2024.

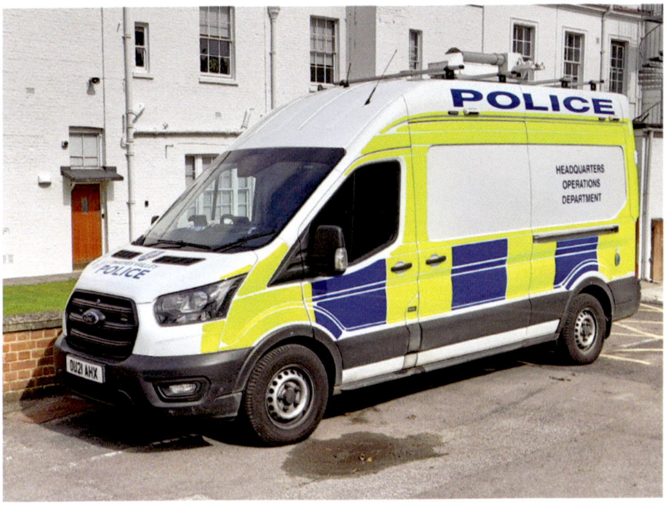

Seen at the TVP's Training Centre at Sulhamstead during the 2023 open day was the latest vehicle with the Headquarters Operations Department at Kidlington. OU21 AHX (2021) is a Ford Transit 350 Leader Ecoblue high-roof van fitted with a roof-rack and a folding telescopic light-mast.

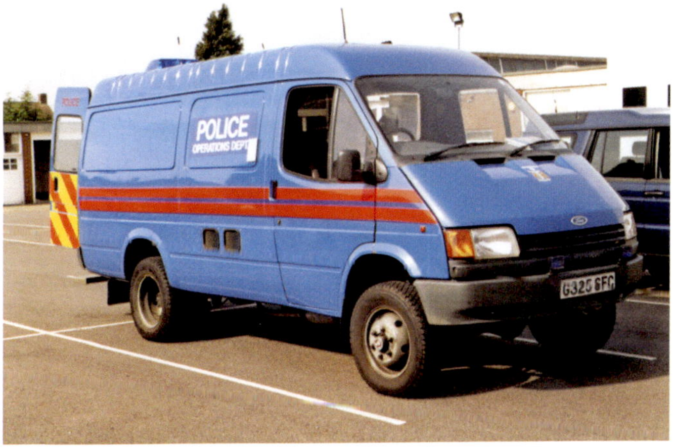

Seen at TVP's HQ in Kidlington in 2002 was one of the few non-white-liveried marked vehicles in the fleet. G325 SFC (1989) is a Ford Transit LWB van fitted with a four wheel-drive system by County Tractors of Knighton in Powys in Mid Wales. The vehicle was used by the Operations Department at HQ for over ten years, attending many crime scenes and serious incidents. It was replaced by an Iveco Daily high-roof van.

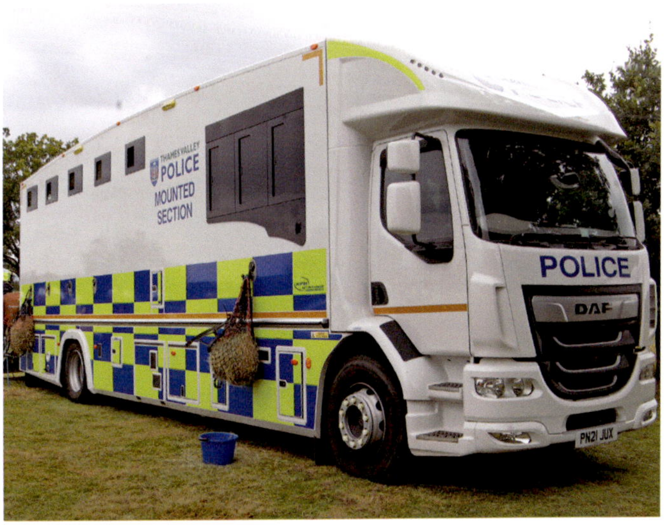

TVP's Mounted Section is based in the north-east of the force area at Milton Keynes Police Station, which is one of the largest stations in the Thames Valley. The newest horsebox in the fleet, PN21 JUX (2021), was built in Lancashire – the Daf LF chassis/cab was built in Leyland and the horsebox body built by KPH near Preston. The vehicle has stalls for five horses, a cab for their riders and low-level lockers for the stowage of equipment. Metal loops along the sides of the body allow feed nets to be hung.

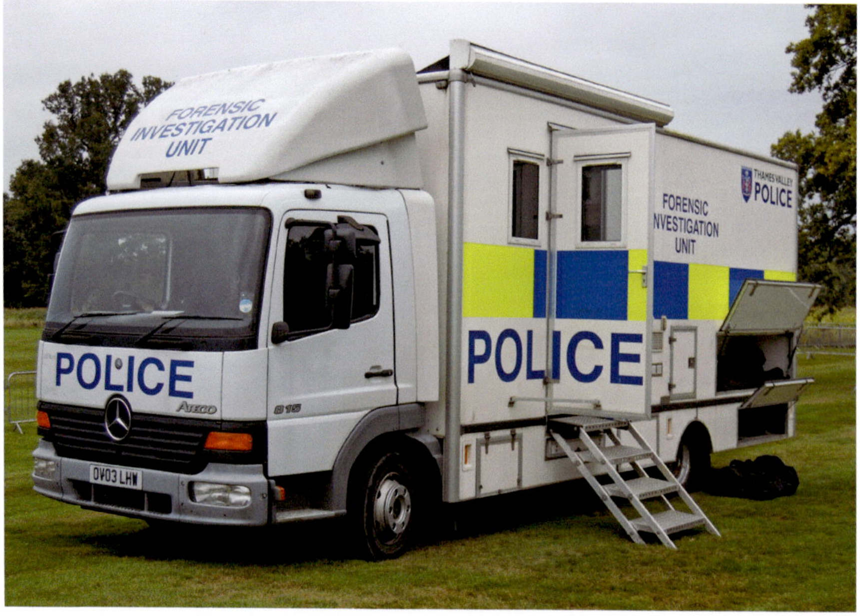

TVP has a number of Vauxhall Vivaro vans used by Crime Scene Investigators (CSI) to carry their equipment. In addition, a Forensic Investigation Unit was purchased to support the CSIs at major crime scenes. OV03 LHW (2003) is a Mercedes Atego 815 chassis fitted with a purpose-built body and an awning. It was on display at the open day at the TVP's Training Centre at Sulhamstead in 2011.

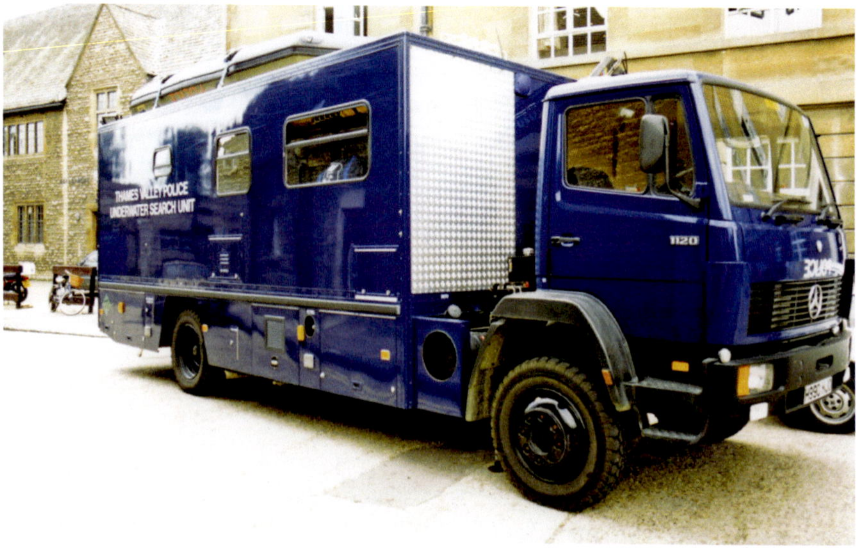

On display outside St Aldate's Police Station in Oxford was TVP's then brand-new Underwater Search Unit. H990 HJO (1991) was built by Locomotors of Andover on a Mercedes 1120 chassis and fitted with a Hiab 020 crane behind the cab and a light-mast at the rear. A wide range of diving equipment was stowed internally and a Zodiac inflatable boat carried on the roof. A few years later, the USU was repainted white and later replaced by a larger Mercedes Atego-based unit.

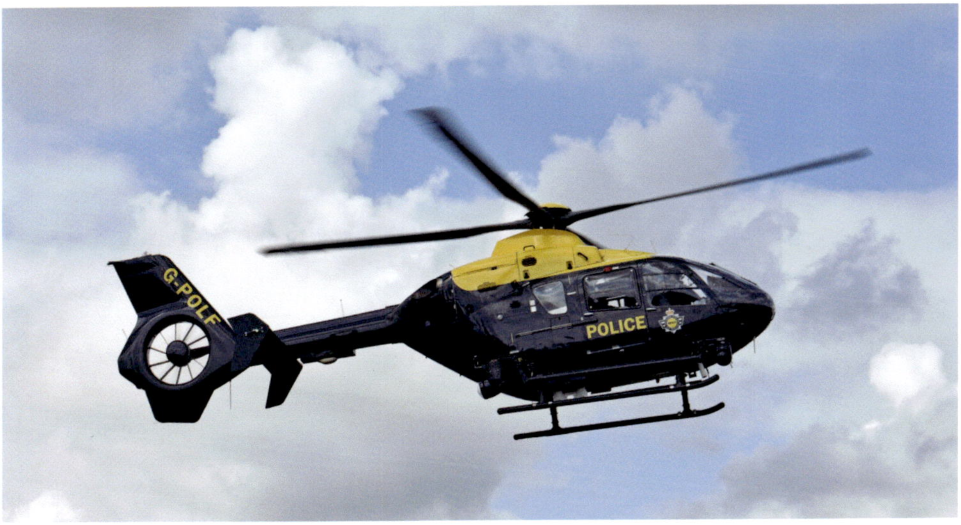

The TVP Air Support Unit was established at Oxford Airport in Kidlington in 1982, operating an Aerospatiale AS350B Squirrel helicopter, before relocating to RAF Abingdon, then returning to Oxford Airport and re-equipping with a MBB Bo-105, relocating again to RAF Benson, using an Aerospatiale AS355F1 Twin Squirrel and later an Eurocopter EC135. The Chiltern ASU (with Bedfordshire and Hertfordshire) was formed in 1996, before most police ASUs were merged into the National Police Air Service in 2012. In 2023, NPAS was operating G-POLF (2002), an Eurocopter EC135 (ex-Essex Police) at Benson.

BRITISH TRANSPORT POLICE

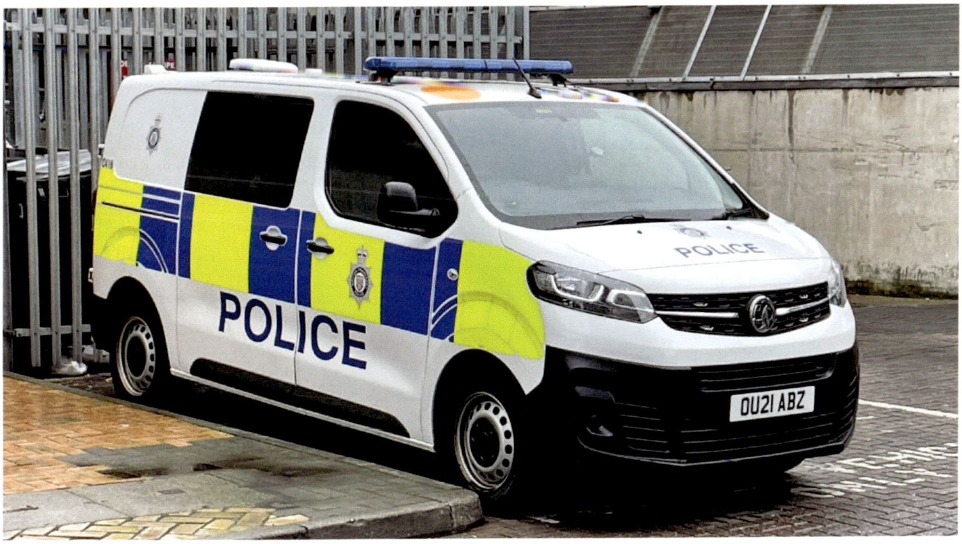

With around 3,000 officers and over 1,000 staff, the British Transport Police (BTP) is one of the largest police forces in Great Britain, policing most railways, some underground systems and some tram systems. In the Thames Valley, BTP officers are based at railway stations in Milton Keynes, Oxford and Reading. This 2021 Vauxhall Vivaro cell van was seen at Reading railway station in Berkshire. (Photo: Gethin Roberts)

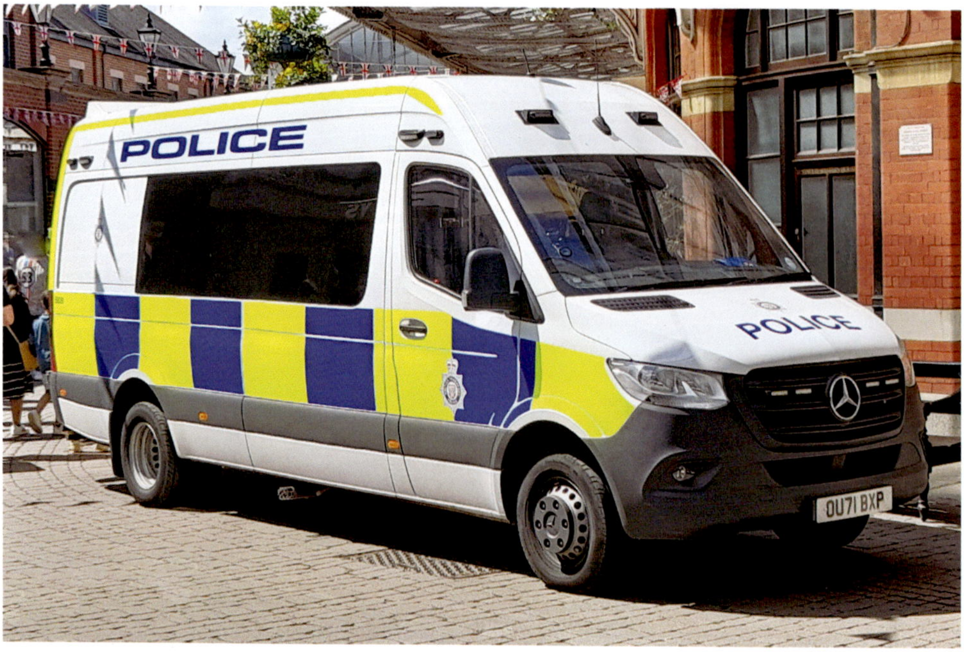

The day after the coronation of King Charles III in May 2023, an open air concert was held on the East Lawn of Windsor Castle, attended by several thousand people, many of whom travelled by train to Windsor and Eton Central railway station. OU71 BXP (2022), a Mercedes Sprinter LWB high-roof personnel carrier, was being used by BTP's Search Team.

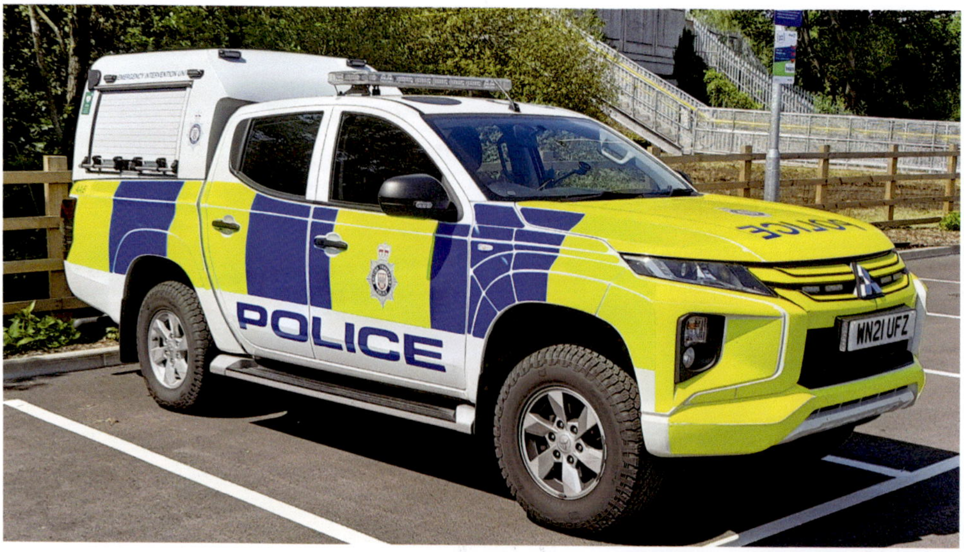

On the first day of passenger services in May 2023, a visitor to the new Green Park railway station in the south of Reading was the Wessex Route Emergency Intervention Unit based at Guildford in Surrey. Crewed by a BTP Police Constable and a Network Rail Mobile Operations Manager, the EIU is equipped to respond to urgent calls affecting railway infrastructure that require the attendance of both BTP and Network Rail. WN21 UFZ (2021) is a Mitsubishi L200 4x4 2.2-litre diesel, double cab pick-up truck fitted with a slide-in/out equipment body by Strongs.

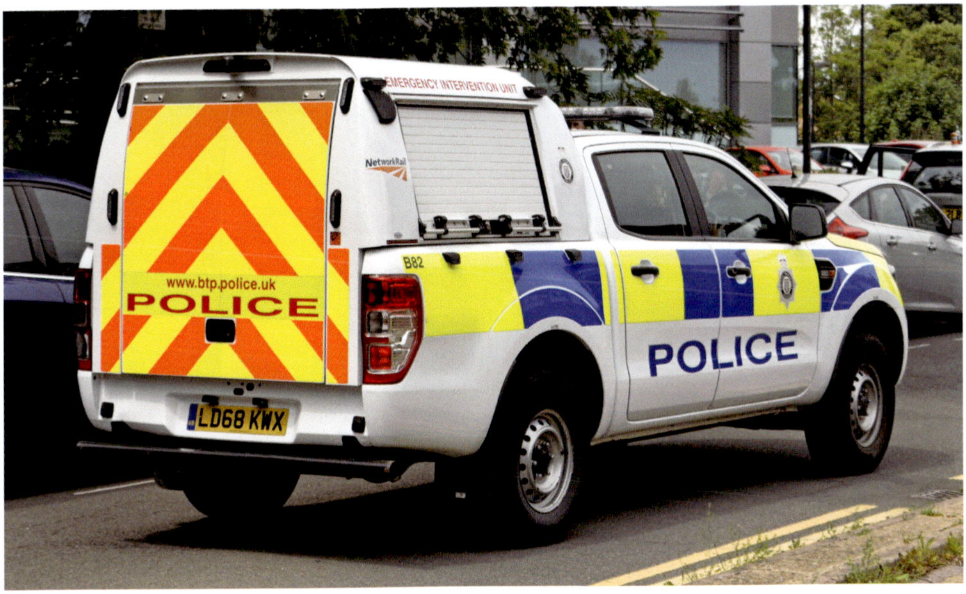

An earlier version of an Emergency Intervention Unit is LD68 KWX (2018), a Ford Ranger 4x4 2.2-litre diesel, double cab pick-up truck also fitted with a slide-in/out equipment body by Strongs. The Western Route EIU, based at Slough, was photographed approaching Maidenhead Police Station in Berkshire in June 2022. At the time of writing, there are six EIUs operating around London on the Anglia, Kent, London North Eastern-East Midlands, Sussex, Wessex and Western routes.

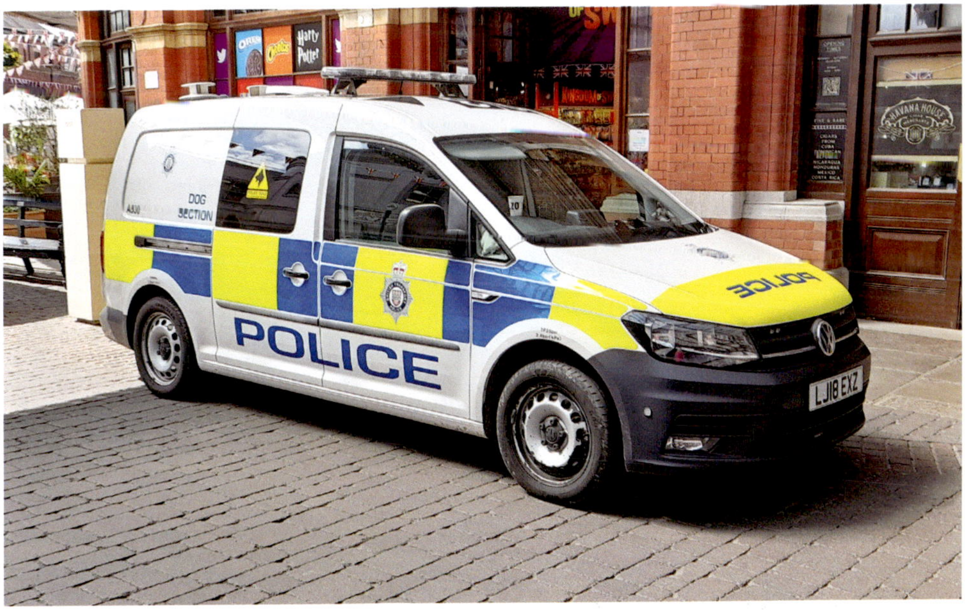

Also seen at Windsor and Eton Central railway station was LJ18 EXZ (2018), a VW Caddy 2.0-litre diesel van fitted with dog cages and sliding side doors. Just visible on the roof above the driver's door is the black triangle symbol, indicating to the crew of a police helicopter or drone operator that the vehicle is a dog unit; the force identifying number for BTP is 93.

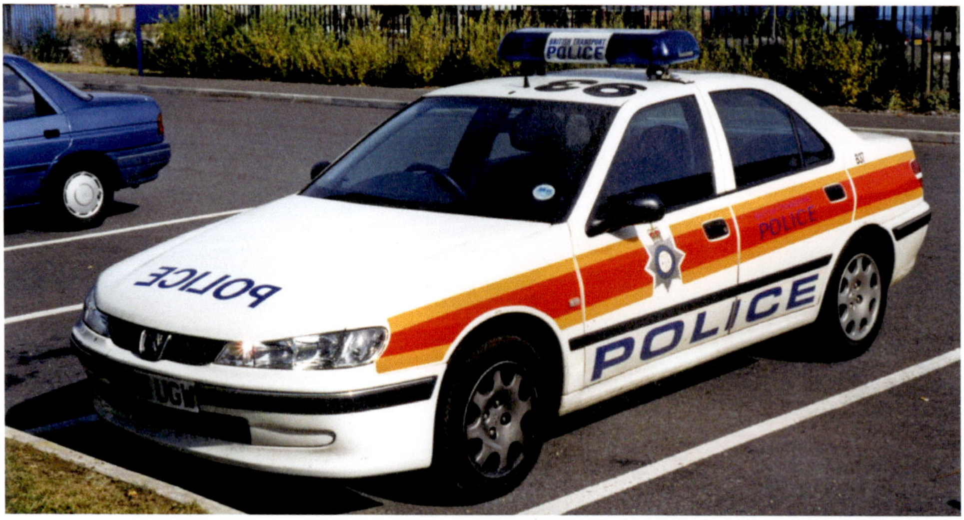

Seen parked outside Abingdon Police Station in 2002 was this BTP Peugeot 406 saloon. W735 UGW (2000) was a 2.0-litre turbo diesel model. The presence of a BTP vehicle in Abingdon is quite unusual as the town's railway station closed in the 1960s. The then freight-only branch line closed in the 1980s, having been used for car trains loaded with MG sports cars built at the factory in Abingdon which closed in 1980, the former main gate area of which is now occupied by the town's police station.

CIVIL NUCLEAR CONSTABULARY/UKAEA CONSTABULARY

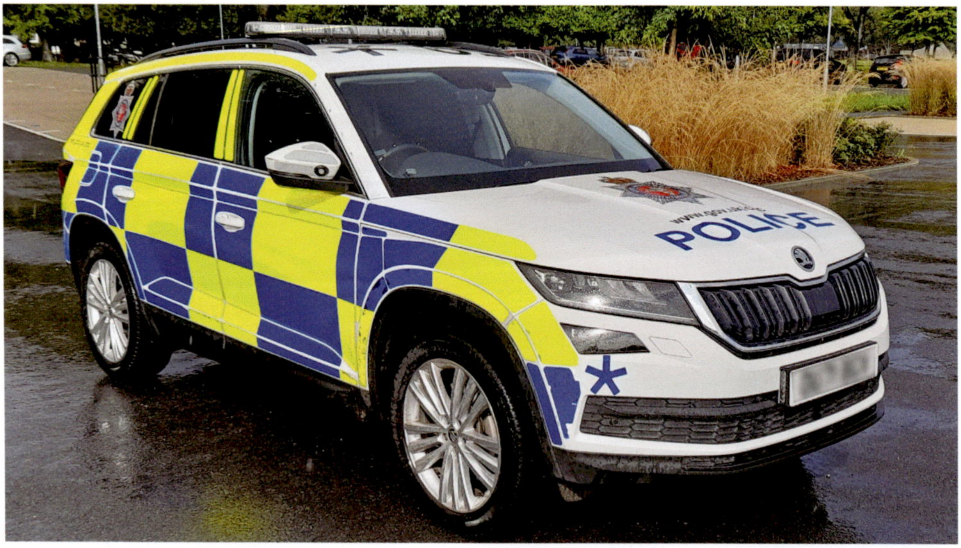

The Civil Nuclear Constabulary was formed in 2005, replacing the United Kingdom Atomic Energy Authority Constabulary. With its headquarters located at Culham Campus in Oxfordshire, the force of around 1600 personnel is responsible for the armed protection of several civil nuclear facilities (including operating nuclear power stations) and Special Nuclear Materials on site and in transit. The Operational Policing Unit at Harwell Campus, also in Oxfordshire, has this 2021 Skoda Kodiaq 4x4 ARV. The force identifying number for CNC is 59.

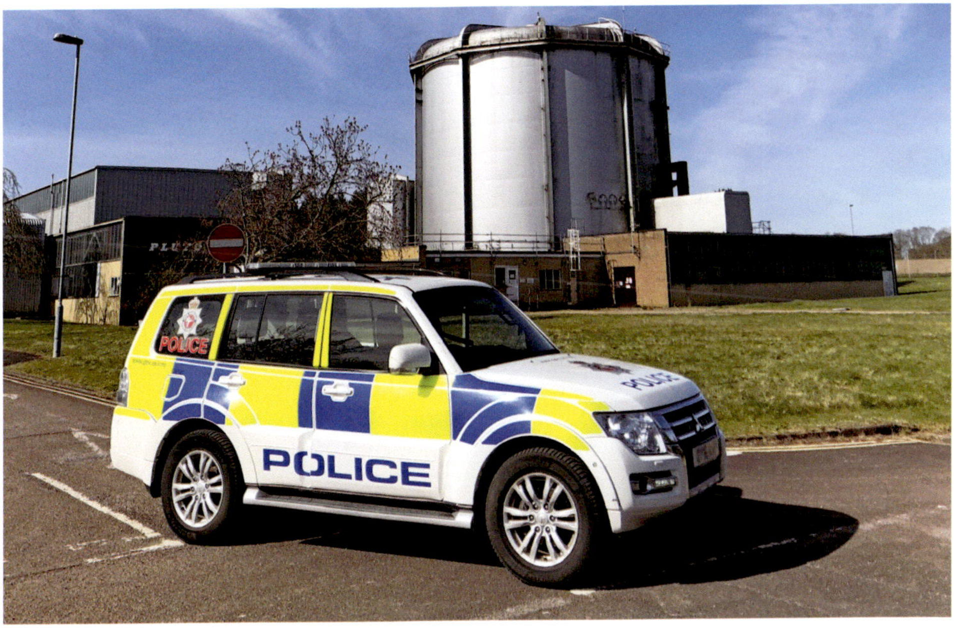

The Harwell Campus is based on the former RAF Harwell airfield (used in support of the D-Day landings). In 1946, Harwell became the site of the Atomic Energy Research Establishment, which was home to the first nuclear reactor in Western Europe, named GLEEP. The location is now a multi-disciplinary advanced research and business centre containing a small nuclear-licensed site. Seen in front of the decommissioned PLUTO Materials Testing Reactor is a Mitsubishi Shogun 4x4 ARV. (Photo: Richard Jones – CNC)

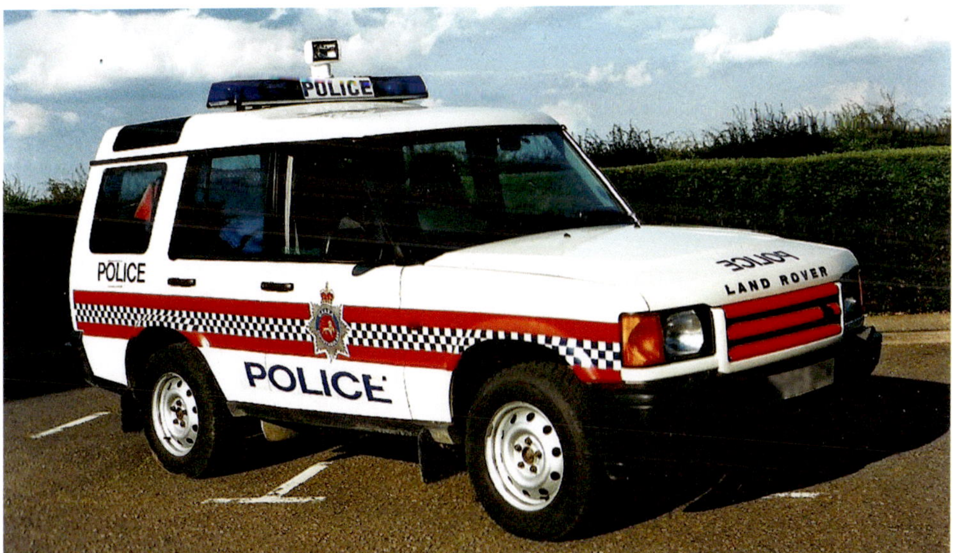

Seen at Harwell in 2002 was this 2000 Land Rover Discovery Td5 4x4 ARV. Based at Sellafield in Cumbria (the UK's largest nuclear site), it was temporarily reallocated to Harwell for a few months to increase armed response capability following the 9/11 terrorist attacks in the USA in September 2001.

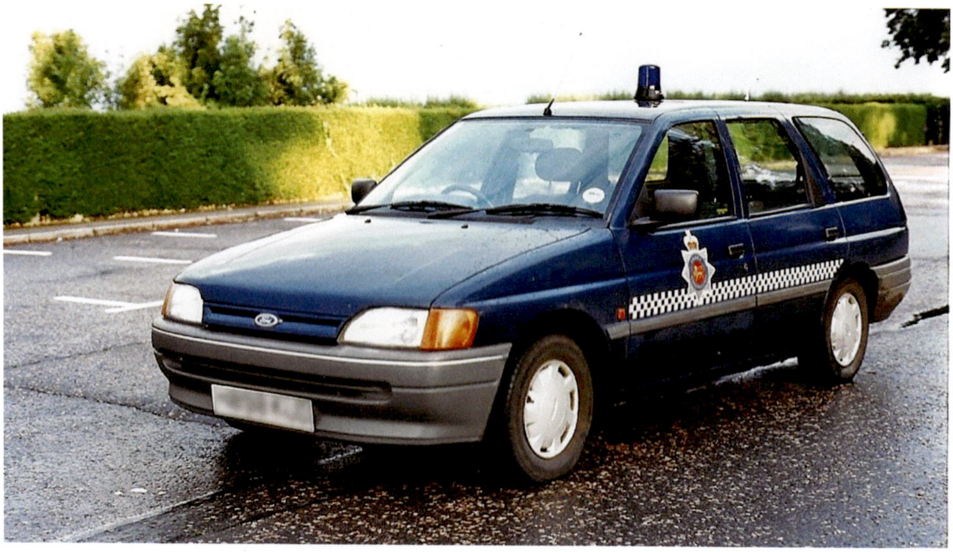

The UKAEA Constabulary was formed in 1955 with headquarters in London and Risley (Cheshire); the headquarters relocated to Culham in the late 1990s. In the 1980s and 1990s, many of the Constabulary's vehicles were dark blue with white and blue cheque stripes. Seen at Harwell in the mid-1990s was this 1991 Ford Escort Mk.5 1.8-litre diesel estate. This vehicle finished its career at the Winfrith site in Dorset in 2002.

MINISTRY OF DEFENCE POLICE

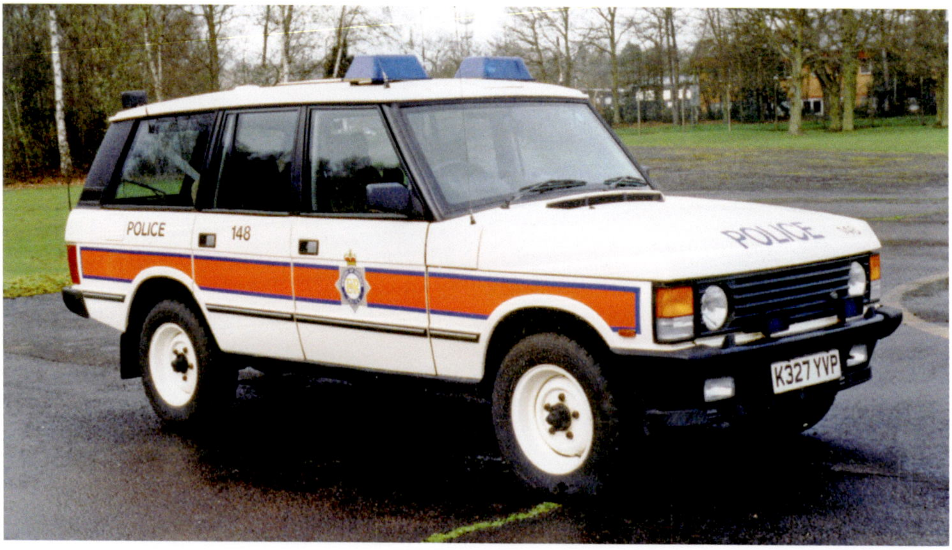

During the 1980s and 1990s, the MDP operated a small fleet of armoured Range Rovers, converted by MacNeillie, for use by their Special Escort Group; they were mainly used to escort convoys carrying Defence Nuclear Materials in support of the UK's nuclear deterrent. K327 YVP (1992) was photographed outside Atomic Weapons Establishment Aldermaston in 1998, before it was re-liveried in Battenberg. Due to the extra weight of the armour, the horizontally split rear doors had to be modified to open vertically.

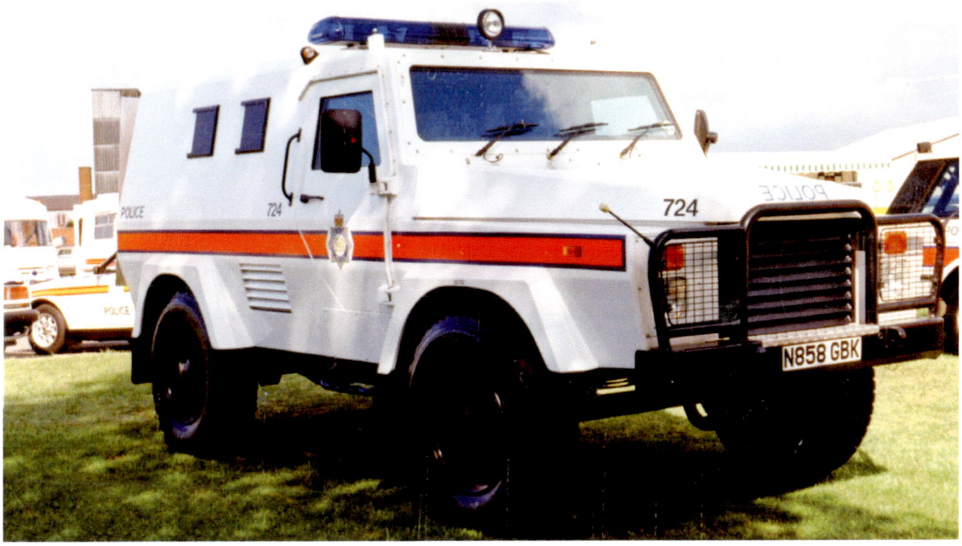

In 1996, the MDP bought four armoured vehicles for use at AWE Aldermaston in Berkshire. Built on heavy, four-wheel-drive chassis by Glover Webb, they could carry several armed police officers. Then brand new, fleet number 724 made the 100-mile journey from Berkshire to Essex to take part in the MDP's 25th anniversary open day at their then headquarters at the former USAF airfield at Wethersfield. The MDP's HQ is now located at RAF Wyton in Cambridgeshire.

ROYAL MILITARY POLICE

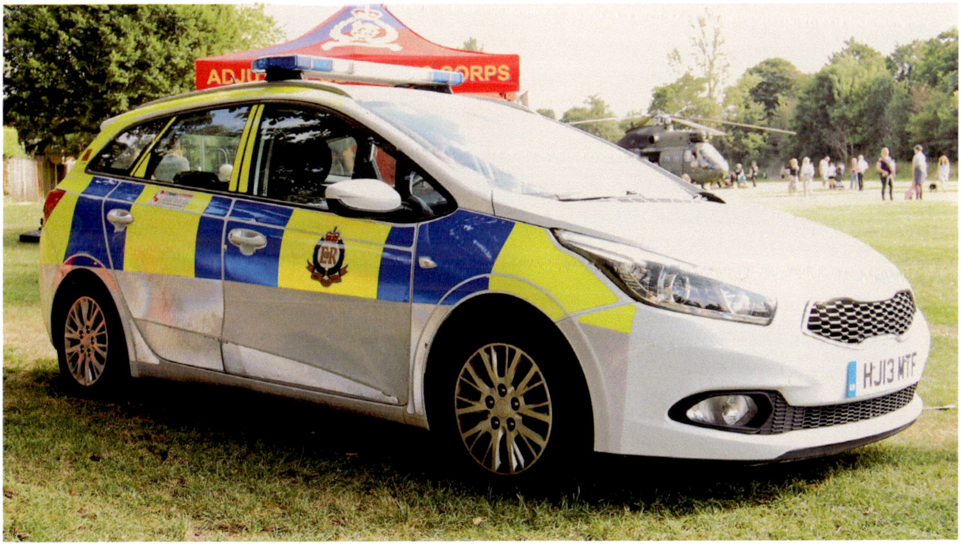

The Royal Military Police provides policing and support to the British Army in the UK and wherever it is deployed overseas, including policing personnel of all three armed forces during peace-time and conflicts. Taking part in an armed forces event in Wallingford in 2017 was this second generation Kia Cee'd hatchback, HJ13 MTF (2013). Just visible in the background is a Puma helicopter from nearby RAF Benson; three Pumas took part in a farewell tour of the UK in March 2025.

UNITED STATES AIR FORCE SECURITY POLICE

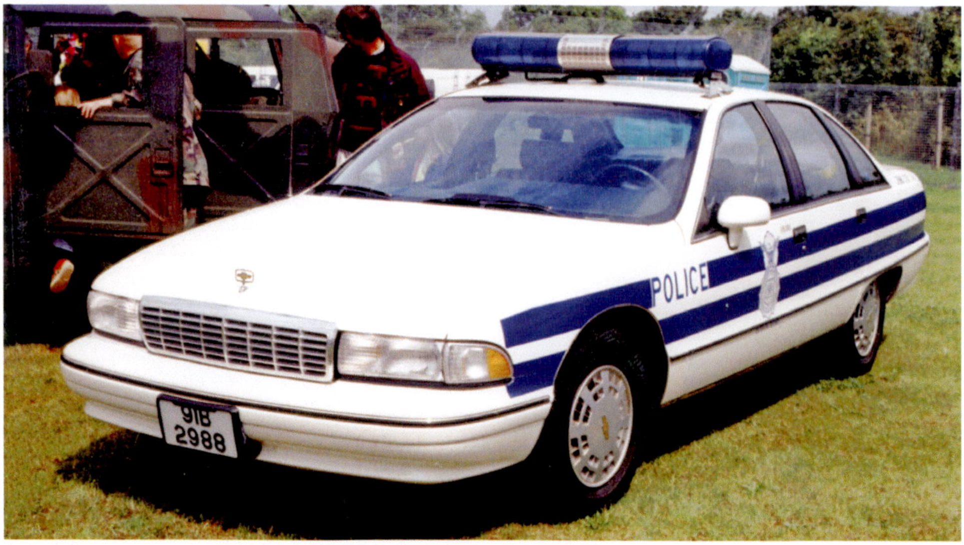

Some of the non-TVP vehicles taking part in the June 1993 open day at the then new Traffic Base and Vehicle Workshops in Bicester, Oxfordshire, were American-built vehicles from the United States Air Force Security Police (USAF SP) based at the nearby RAF Upper Heyford. 91 B 2988 is a 1991, fourth generation Chevrolet Caprice 9C1. Earlier versions of the Caprice were also used by the USAF SP at Upper Heyford. The USAF SP became the USAF Security Forces in 1997.

ROYAL AIR FORCE POLICE

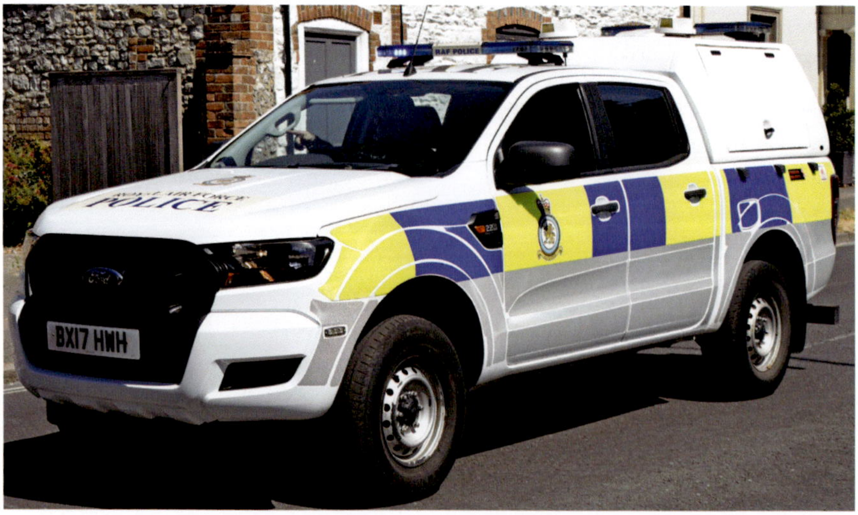

In August 2022, personnel from RAF Benson marched through Wallingford to exercise the Freedom of Wallingford, the first parade having taken place in 1957. RAF Police and armed TVP officers escorted the march through the town centre. One of the RAFP vehicles escorting the RAF band and personnel was BX17 HWH (2017), a Ford Ranger 4x4, double cab, fitted with a Truckman hard-top over the load-bed. This vehicle has large black RAF lettering on the cab roof.

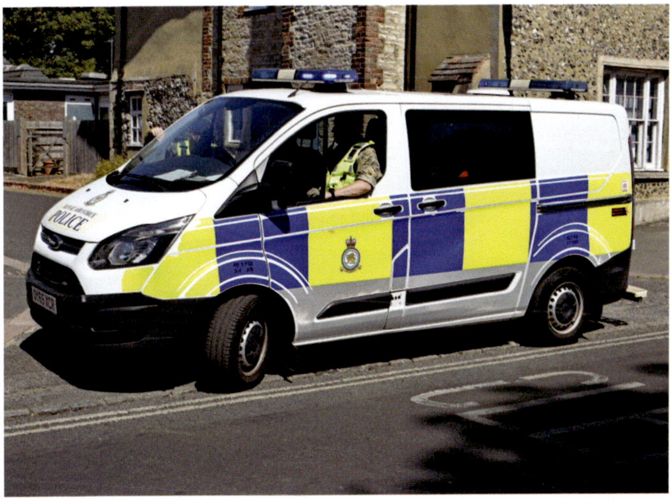

Another of the RAFP vehicles from Benson was this Ford Transit SWB combi van, OY65 XCR (2015). The RAF Police headquarters is located at RAF Honington in Suffolk. Phase One training (basic recruit training) is a ten-week course at RAF Halton in Buckinghamshire. This is followed by Phase Two training (RAF Police Initial Course), which is a twenty-two-week course at the Defence School of Policing and Guarding at Southwick Park in Hampshire.

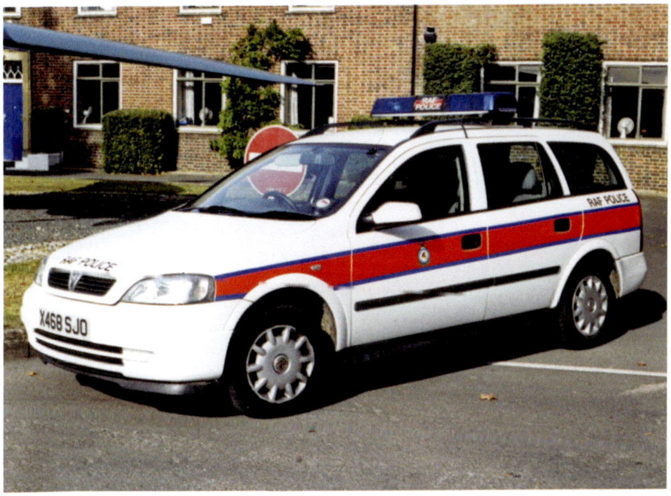

Seen at RAF Benson in the mid-2000s, this RAFP patrol car was parked at the main gate. X468 SJO is a 2000 Vauxhall Astra diesel estate. Visible in the background is the wing of the gate guardian, a replica of a Supermarine Spitfire of No. 1 Photographic Reconnaissance Unit, which was based at RAF Benson during the Second World War.

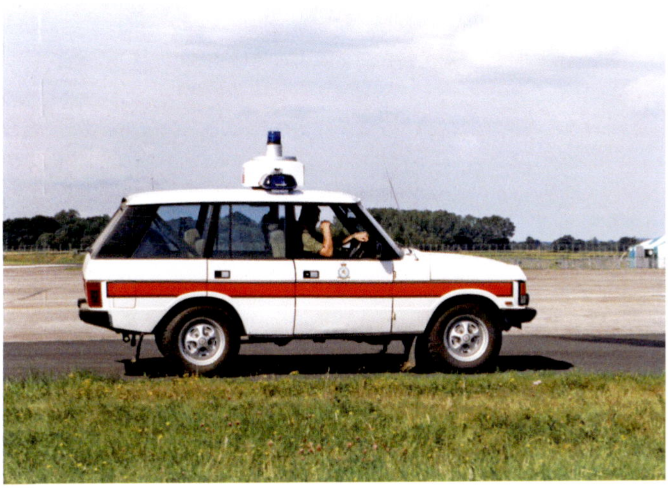

In addition to a large fleet of Land Rovers, the RAF Police operated a small number of Range Rovers. This RAFP Range Rover was seen at an event at RAF Brize Norton in Oxfordshire in the mid-1990s. At that time the Range Rover is likely to have been based with the RAF Provost and Security Squadron at the former RAF Rudloe Manor in Wiltshire, before the squadron moved to RAF Henlow in Bedfordshire. (Photo: the late Ray Roberts)

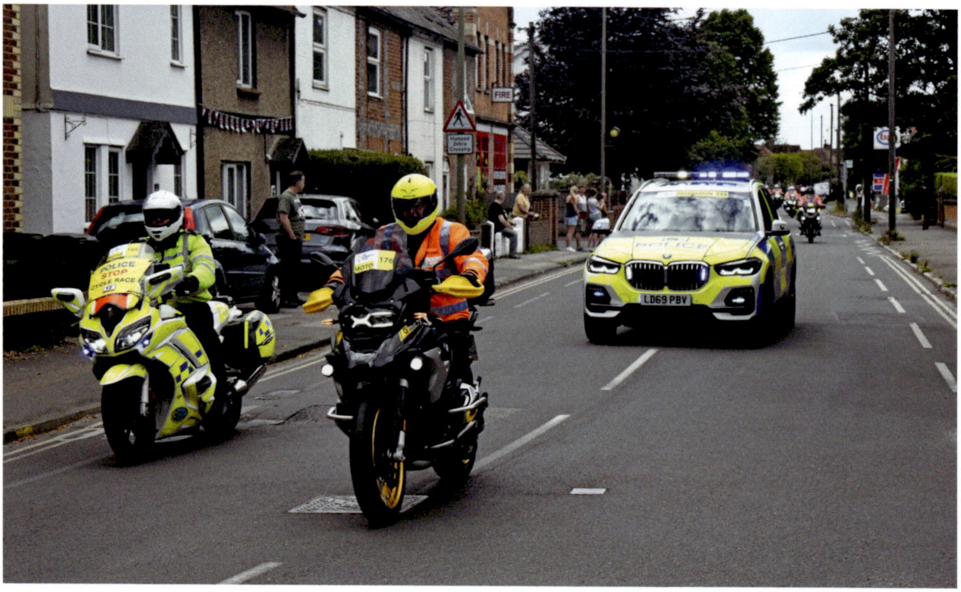

Although impossible to convey in a book, the sight and sound of approximately thirty motorcycles passing Wallingford Fire Station (which celebrated its 100th anniversary in 2024) ahead of the riders taking part in the June 2022 Women's Tour of Britain cycle race was impressive! The motorcyclists came from the civilian NEG and various police forces, including Avon & Somerset, Gwent, Suffolk and West Yorkshire. The BMW X5 4x4, LD69 PBV (2019), is a BMW demonstrator (fleet number BMW 679).

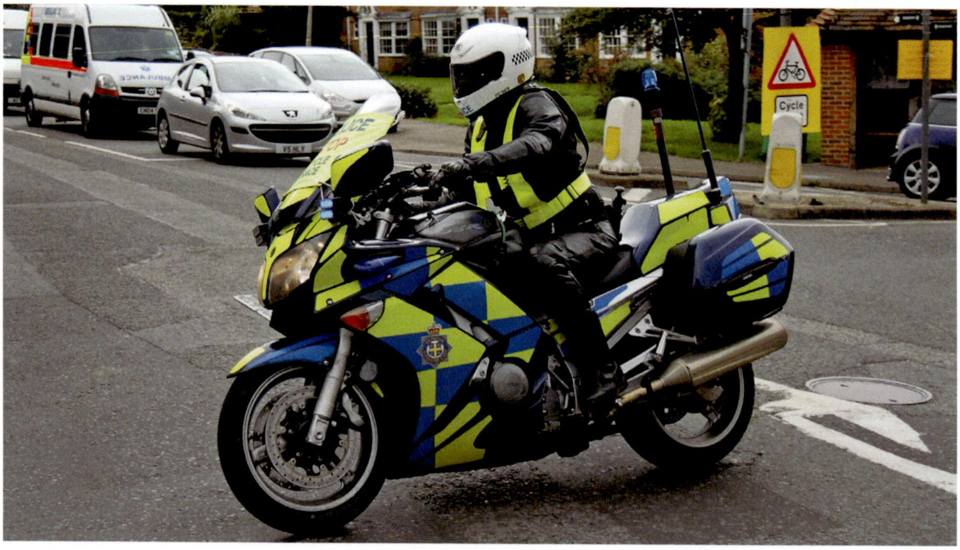

The 2008 men's Tour of Britain cycle race took place in September of that year. The second stage was 145 km (90 miles) from Milton Keynes to Newbury. Having just crossed the River Thames, this Durham Constabulary Yamaha FJR motorcycle is crossing the A329 and starting the short but steep climb of Streatley Hill in Berkshire. Streatley Hill was a category two climb in the King of the Mountains jersey competition, with a distance of 1.3 km (0.8 miles), a gradient of almost 10 per cent (1 in 10) and a vertical change in height of almost 110 metres (361 feet).

Conclusion

Hopefully, the photographs in this book have been able to illustrate a good variety of the vehicles operated by a wide range of emergency services and organisations across the Thames Valley. Also, the text and captions have provided useful information and items of interest to both those with and without a detailed knowledge of the emergency services and their vehicles.

Most of the vehicles featured are used by emergency services personnel working on the front line but we must also remember the staff behind the scenes, including Control Room operators, medical staff, fleet managers, vehicle mechanics, equipment technicians, administrators, press officers, instructors, emergency planners and many more, be they uniformed or non-uniformed and whether they are permanent staff, part-time, on-call or volunteers.

As with similar publications on the emergency services or transport in general, some aspects of a book of this type are likely to be out of date when it is published, in that some current vehicles featured will have been replaced and organisational changes will have taken place. At the time of writing, new vehicles were being issued to some of the emergency services, including the NHS ambulance service's Hazardous Area Response Teams, the British Army's Explosive Ordnance Disposal troops and Network Rail's incident response teams. In addition, Rewley Road Fire Station in Oxford is scheduled for replacement, the Thames Valley Police is undergoing reorganisation and the Civil Nuclear Constabulary will take on the armed protection of three coastal gas terminals.

Finally, all emergency services personnel deserve our thanks and support.

Geraint H. Roberts
Wallingford, Oxfordshire, July 2025

Acknowledgements

A very big thank you to all of the firefighters, police officers, paramedics, technicians, mechanics, support staff, receptionists, administrators, managers, senior officers, medical staff, charity workers, military personnel, and railways and highways staff who have allowed visits, moved vehicles for photography, demonstrated equipment, answered numerous questions and provided information.

In particular, I am very grateful to the following personnel from the emergency services and other organisations for their help with this project: AWE Aldermaston – Nicole Targett (Media & PR), British Transport Police – Corrie David (Media Relations), Buckinghamshire F&RS – Communication Team, Civil Nuclear Constabulary – Daniel Riddle (Corporate Communications) and Sergeants Richard and Luke (Harwell), Lowland Rescue Oxfordshire – Marcus Nurton (Chair), Ministry of Defence – Panay Triantafillides (Defence Imagery), National Highways – Jo Grey (Customer Strategy & Communications Directorate) and Ross and Jake (Chieveley Outstation), Network Rail – Chris O'Connell (Wales & Western), Oxfordshire F&RS – Rob MacDougall (CFO), Royal Air Force Benson and Brize Norton – Media and Engagement, HQ Air Command – Air Policy Secretariat; tiny hamlets, isolated farms and country houses. Royal Berkshire F&RS – Mark Antell (Communications and Engagement Team), South Central Ambulance Service – David Gallagher (External Relations) and driving instructors (Newbury Education Centre), Thames Valley Police – Brent Jones (Corporate Communications); and TRL – Penny While (Marketing). Also, all of the landowners who have given permission for photographs taken on their land to be published in this book.

Thanks also go to many other people and volunteers, including members of the Police Vehicle Enthusiasts Club, who have arranged visits to the emergency services or have organised and staffed open days, community safety events, charity events and historic vehicle rallies.

Additionally, thank you to the following current and past members of The Fire Brigade Society for organising visits to numerous fire stations and many other locations; for their help, advice, encouragement, enthusiasm, ideas, suggestions, inspiration and willingness to share information and photographs, which have helped me to develop my interest, knowledge and appreciation of the emergency services over almost forty years: Ivan Barefield, Simon Bartlett, Dave Boulter MBE, Nigel Crompton, Colin Dunford, the late Charles Keevil, the late Roger Mardon, Roger Pearce, Simon Pearce, the late David Riggs, Ian Scott, Bob Smith, Martin Smith, Mike Smith, Gavin Stewart, John Thompson and the late Mike Williams.

Thanks also go to Nick Grant and the team at Amberley Publishing for their guidance.

Finally, many thanks go to my family (my wife Gillian, my son Gethin, my daughter Gwenifer, my brother Richard, my mum Carol and my late dad Ray) for their support and patience with many photo stops on family trips and visits to open days and events and taking photos for me when I have been elsewhere.